Mind Gone Astray

Mind Gone Astray

Wayne Kallio

iUniverse, Inc.
New York   Bloomington

Mind Gone Astray

Copyright © 2009 by Wayne Kallio

All rights reserved. No part of this book may be used or reproduced by any means, graphic, electronic, or mechanical, including photocopying, recording, taping or by any information storage retrieval system without the written permission of the publisher except in the case of brief quotations embodied in critical articles and reviews.

iUniverse books may be ordered through booksellers or by contacting:

iUniverse
1663 Liberty Drive
Bloomington, IN 47403
www.iuniverse.com
1-800-Authors (1-800-288-4677)

Because of the dynamic nature of the Internet, any Web addresses or links contained in this book may have changed since publication and may no longer be valid. The views expressed in this work are solely those of the author and do not necessarily reflect the views of the publisher, and the publisher hereby disclaims any responsibility for them.

ISBN: 978-1-4401-2116-6 (pbk)
ISBN: 978-1-4401-2117-3 (ebk)

Printed in the United States of America

iUniverse rev. date: 2/19/2009

Foreword

This is a true story. Only the names of individuals and places have been changed. The setting is deliberately left vague in order to retain the story's universal appeal. In today's world, psychotic disorders of various kinds seem to be more rampant (one in four will suffer from some form of mental illness in his or her lifetime), or perhaps we have just recently begun to recognize them for what they truly are. Most of us have a loved one or a friend, or know of someone who suffers from a mental illness, yet few of us know how to respond to such a person or situation.

In the past, individuals with schizophrenia, for example, were considered "crazy" and were institutionalized, usually for the rest of their lives. Thought disorders such as schizophrenia have been distorted by stories such as the early *Dr. Jekyll and Mr. Hyde*, and by more recent ones such as *One Flew Over the Cuckoo's Nest* and *Silence of the Lambs*, to name only a few. Modern research into mental illness has lagged far behind that of research into physical illness. Over the past two decades, however, great strides have been made in both diagnosing and treating mental illness; public awareness has been heightened; and governments have begun to fund research and development for mental illnesses at an unprecedented rate.

In spite of this, knowledge and understanding of mental illness (compared to that of physical illness) remains in the dark ages. The one constant defining characteristic of schizophrenia, which this story is about, is the profound feeling of incomprehensibility and inaccessibility that sufferers of the disease provoke in other people. Because of this, the stigma of "crazy" remains. To help eliminate this stigma is one of the main objectives in writing this book.

The story deliberately contains circular, repetitious patterns because that's how it happened. It is a common characteristic of many psychoses. Such is the nature of schizophrenia. Feel it. Feel the déjà vu, the frustration, the impatience, the helplessness, the desperate grasping for comprehension, the angst, the despair, the shattered hopes. But feel, too, the depth of faith and love, and above all, the hope that intermittently bursts forth like the first crocuses in spring. There are shafts of light piercing the darkness.

The purpose of this story, then, is to help bring enlightenment of a schizophrenia-like psychosis to the common citizen so that the incomprehensible may gradually become comprehensible, so that labels such as "crazy" and "off her rocker" will disappear as understanding grows, and so that mental illness will come to be accepted as an illness not unlike a physical illness. It is a cry for awareness and understanding.

CONTENTS

Chapter 1: The Beginning 1
Chapter 2: Name Branding 8
Chapter 3: The Unforgettable Ride 13
Chapter 4: ER 18
Chapter 5: The Dungeon 27
Chapter 6: Roller-Coaster Ride 39
Chapter 7: ECT 49
Chapter 8: Passages Home 56
Chapter 9: Home Again! 82
Chapter 10: Back in the Dungeon 96
Chapter 11: Déjà vu 112
Chapter 12: Episodic Nightmare 123
Chapter 13: A Glimmer of Light 138
Chapter 14: Compulsions and Obsessions 146
Chapter 15: Crisis 171
Chapter 16: We've Been Here Before 177
Chapter 17: What Next? 187
Chapter 18: Psychotic Systems and People 194
Chapter 19: Still Roller Coasting 208
Chapter 20: Will It Ever End? 216
Chapter 21: Kiss of Death 221
Chapter 22: Hope Springs Eternal 232

Chapter 1: The Beginning

It had happened just that suddenly. Or at least I thought it had. I had come home from work and had expected my wife to be preparing supper as usual. But the kitchen was empty, no supper cooking.

"Where are you?" I had called. No response. Then, suddenly, she was there before me, pale, eyes wide with apprehension.

"I was upstairs," she said. *"I was hiding because they were out there in a black car waiting for me. Is Dr. Naipaul OK? His wife shot him and he's in the General Hospital. But lucky he repented a long time ago, so if he dies he'll go to heaven. He said he'd come to church if he can. Mrs. Naipaul sent two hit men in a black limousine to get us last night, but they eluded the police and got away. The police watched our house for five hours today. They had tasers on them. But the guys never came back."*

I had been flabbergasted. What on earth was she talking about? "What's wrong, hon?" I had blurted out. "You're not making any sense. Have you taken too many painkillers or something?" I recalled the one time she had—or at least I had thought she had—and how scared I had been as she babbled on incoherently. Something about guys in trench coats, having to put dead bolts on the doors, her father being in heaven, and on and on. But that had been a long time ago, perhaps a couple of years already. I had forgotten all about it.

"I haven't taken anything. *I'm just telling you what happened so you'll know to watch out for them. They have bombs, too. Flutter bombs. You can't even hear them because they flutter down so silently.* I'm glad you're home. I was worried about you."

"Honey, you're not making any sense. Dr. Naipaul is my heart doctor in the city. Why would he be here? And he's never come to our church. And what's all this about hit men and black limousines and police with tasers? There's something wrong. You're hallucinating. We've got to get you to the hospital right away!"

"I'm not hallucinating, and I'm not going to any hospital," she had said vehemently. *"But we have to be careful so they don't get into the house by being invisible."*

And that's how it had begun. She had refused to leave the house, no matter how much I pleaded with her. I slept little that night, lying awake, hoping and praying that she had just screwed up in taking her antidepressants and her painkillers for her fibromyalgia. It would be OK in the morning, I thought.

But it wasn't. She came downstairs in tears. *"Heavenly Father is trying me,"* she lamented over and over. *"Don't keep testing me, please,"* she pleaded, fists clenched, tears running down her cheeks. But then, suddenly, *"He wants to bless us. He may send me to heaven yet tonight."* Big happy smile. *"He just pushes a button and it lets one in, or else he'll just blow them away."*

That's when I knew for sure. Something was desperately wrong. This was no mix-up in medications. I didn't know what it was, but it was a lot more serious than that. Now I was really afraid. I had to get her to a doctor. "Come, darling, let's just go to Emergency at the hospital. Dr. Naipaul is likely there," I lied guiltily. "You can talk to him and see if they've stopped his bullet wound from bleeding." She acquiesced and went willingly.

Of course she was admitted. It didn't take Dr. McRae, our family doctor, long to see that he was dealing with a sick, sick patient. He was one of those sharp young doctors from South Africa, the best one Riverview had ever had. We had been going to him for a long time, and I trusted him.

"What day of the week is this?"

"Wednesday."

"No, actually it's Thursday. But that's OK."

"I get mixed up sometimes because they start the week on Sunday now, and not on Monday as they did in the Bible. God rested after his work, not before!"

"Do you know what month this is?"

"Of course! I'm not that stupid! It's May."

"You're right. I don't think you're stupid, but sometimes we all get our days and dates and months mixed up, so it's a standard question that we ask. Now, count backward, by threes, starting at twenty."

"Twenty, seventeen, fourteen, ten, seven, four, one."

"Can you name the seven continents?"

"Africa, Eastern and Western Europe, but they call it the European Union now so maybe it's one continent instead of two. Then there's Asia and Antarctica and North and Central and South America. Oh, and Australia, I almost forgot that one. Did I get that right? I've been out of school for a long time!"

"Well, that's pretty close. Are you worried about anything?"

"*Only about my platelets sticking. They're only thirty-eight over forty-four and if they go below thirty I'll die.*"

"I see. We need to have a look at that and see what's causing it. You seem to have a bit of trouble concentrating, too, and I think we should admit you, just to take some blood tests to see that everything is all right there. We might have to adjust your antidepressant medication, too."

I saw through Dr. McRae's ruse right away, but it satisfied her, at least for the moment, and it was achieving what I knew was necessary—hospital admission and professional care.

"Kaija has some kind of psychosis," Dr. McRae told me confidentially later. "That may sound scary, but since it's come on so quickly, I think we can treat it with antipsychotics and she'll likely be free of it in two or three months."

I sighed with uneasy relief and went to school. I wished my English teaching job was not so far away, but if necessary, I could be back in Riverview within a half hour by pushing it. At least I knew that now Kaija was safe and in good hands.

As I drove to school, I recalled the unnerving incident that had occurred just five weeks into our marriage. I was still farming then, and I had gone late one evening to load our one-ton International with seed oats. Kaija had come along to help.

"While you clean up around the granary door, I'll lower the grain auger," Kaija offered. But as she was lowering it, the handle slipped and it hit her in the mouth with a *thwack*.

In just a few minutes Kaija's mouth was swollen so that it was just a mass of red flesh. She sobbed uncontrollably, and it seemed that her legs would not hold her upright.

"Are you all right?" I asked, as I held her close.

"I don't know. I'm dizzy and weak and my front teeth are loose. I'm sorry, hon. Don't be mad at me. I shouldn't have gone with you …"

"Nonsense! Accidents happen. But I'm taking you to the doctor right away."

That should have been the end of the episode; the doctor had examined Kaija, given her some Tylenol, and sent her home to rest. But when I came in for my noon lunch the next day, I found Kaija in tears.

"I don't know what's wrong. When I went to feed the chicks, I had to stop and get my breath after every few steps. Now I can't even think straight," she cried. "I don't know what to get you for lunch."

"Don't cry, hon. It's probably due to the Tylenol; that's a heavy dose he put you on. I'll just make myself a ham sandwich. You go back and lie down."

When I came in for supper, Kaija seemed better. She was up, the swelling had gone down quite a lot, and she seemed OK—that is, until she said, as we were sitting at supper, *"Look at that milk pitcher walk across the table!"*

"That's crazy! It can't possibly move on its own …"

"Yes it can! Look for yourself. See, there it goes again! The

salt and pepper are dancing around, too. And you look like you're in a fog or something ..."

I was frightened out of my wits. What was happening? Kaija had lost it, gone over the edge, or something. Had the blow caused her brain damage? It had to have been severe, for the whole weight of the grain auger was on that handle. In any case, we headed for the doctor's office at once.

"Don't look so frightened" were the doctor's words as he examined her again. "She just has a severe concussion. I'm sorry I didn't notice this the first time. I should have kept her in for observation. But she'll be fine if she takes these pills and just rests for the next four or five days."

Such proved to be the case. My fears lessened day by day as Kaija improved. My relief was immense. Her mind had not been damaged after all! But now, looking back, I shuddered at what I feared could have been the death—or madness—of my wife. It brought tears to my eyes. I was thankful that God had protected her then, and I prayed that he would do so again now.

But I was worried. There was that strange disability that she had been telling my sister about just two weeks ago. Something about not being able to bend properly anymore because five vertebrae in her lower back were fused and she'd have to have surgery so they could encase each vertebra individually in gold plating to prevent further deterioration. It was eerie. My sister sounded mystified and worried about it when she called. I knew that Kaija had X-rays taken during her annual medical a couple of weeks ago, but funny, I thought, that she hadn't mentioned anything to me. And encased in gold? Well, what did I know about modern surgical technique? They put wire mesh stents into hearts, and metal reinforcements of all kinds into broken and worn-out bones nowadays, without even operating, so I guessed anything was possible. But I could not shake off that nagging fear ...

Chapter 2: Name Branding

I got the call at noon, at school. Eileen, the secretary, called me out of my English class, which was a bit unusual.

"I think you should take this call," she said when I got to the office. "It's Susan, the Riverview School secretary, and she said it was important. She sounded kinda worried."

I picked up the phone. "Hello. This is Mr. Koivu."

"You're wife's purse and a bag of notions and such are here at the office, Mr. Koivu. I'm a bit worried because they were found in the parking lot here at the school. I hope they weren't stolen."

"What? What do you mean? How did they get there? She's in the hospital!" My heart sank. Something was dreadfully wrong.

"Oh! I didn't know that. I have no idea how they ended up here. No one has seen Kaija—at least she hasn't been to the library here ... Anyway, you can pick them up at the front desk, when you get back into town after work."

"I'll be there in a half hour," I almost shouted, and slammed the receiver down.

Twenty minutes later, Susan informed me that a student had found Kaija's purse and the bag of belongings tucked away between her car and the hedgerow at the far end of the student parking lot. I was baffled. Had she run away from the hospital? If so, why had she gone there? And where was she now? At home? Wandering the streets somewhere? Back in the hospital? I swiftly drove there.

"Is Kaija here?" I shouted to the nurse at the front desk.

"Yes, she eloped. That's what we call patients who try to get away. But she's back now. Your nephew, Jim, apparently found her sitting in his half-ton in front of their machine shop on the east side of town. She got by us somehow and must have walked all the way over there. That's a long hike. We have her sedated now, as she was really agitated when he brought her back here. Jim had a hard time getting her to come in. If she elopes like that again, you'll have to arrange for someone to sit with her because we don't have an alarm system and we can't watch all the exits all the time."

Even though she was now safe, I felt a cold fear inside. Why had she escaped and gone there? And why on earth had she hidden her purse and belongings in the parking lot? What if ... I dared not complete the thoughts that were thrusting themselves into my mind. I hurried to her room.

"Hi, hon. Are you OK?" I asked as I held her close. She had a haunted look in her eyes and held me tightly. "Why did you leave the hospital and go to the guy's' machine shop?"

"I had to warn them."

"Warn them of what?"

"Of the flutter bombs. They were going to bomb the whole third floor of the shop."

"There is no third floor ..."

"Yes there is. I didn't dare go in so I sat outside in Jim's half-ton and kept watch. Pretty soon Jim came out and found me waiting there so I told him what was going to happen. He said that we'd better get away from there and drove me back here. I wanted to go home but he wouldn't take me there. Are you finished teaching for the day?"

"Yes. But I can't take you home. The doctor wants to take some more blood tests in the morning. Why did you leave your purse in the school parking lot?"

"Because I had two million dollars in it and I was afraid someone would grab my purse from me."

"Oh. OK. But promise me you won't leave the hospital tomorrow, OK? I have to go home and eat now, but I'll come back and visit you in the evening."

I called Jim as soon as I got home. "Yeah. I went to get my socket set from my truck and there she was, just sitting there. I don't know how long she'd been there. I asked her what she wanted and she rambled on about somebody going to bomb our building and that we'd better get out of there. She talked about some kind of floating or fluttering bombs or something. It was weird. I could tell she was wired or something and I knew she had been in the hospital, so I drove her straight back there."

"Thanks, Jim. Yeah, something seems to be wrong with her mind, but the doc doesn't know what yet. But she's a sick girl, that I know."

I worried all through the next day at school. I phoned

the hospital twice, and both times was told that she had again left the hospital on her own but they had noticed and gone after her and brought her back. The second time she had gone three blocks before they caught up to her.

"She's definitely an eloper," the nurse told me when I arrived at the hospital after school. She'll have to have someone with her full-time as long as she's here. We've given her Ativan every three hours to keep her calmed down, as she's pretty agitated otherwise. We had to give her a shot of morphine last night to get her to go to sleep. But that didn't help. She's paced the halls day and night."

She was in the bathroom, talking to herself, when I went to her room. "What are you doing in there so long?" I asked.

"I'm swiping the sink and the toilet seat"

"What do you mean, swiping it?"

She opened the door. "See, I have to wipe everything down like this with a damp face cloth. I have to do it many times a day because of the germs. I had to lie on the floor with my feet against the door this afternoon to keep that guy from coming in here."

"What guy?"

"Just one of those guys that are always slinking around."

"How come you left the hospital again today?"

"Oh, I just went to warn the people, but these stupid nurses always came and made me come back. Did they think I was going to kill myself or something?" I shuddered at that last thought. I couldn't imagine what was going on in her

mind. Yet suddenly she seemed totally rational. "How was school? Did you have to stay late?"

"Just an hour to talk with some parents."

"Were the kids bad?"

"No worse than usual. The grade nines were restless, as alwaysl"

"Will I get out of here tomorrow?"

"I don't know. I'll talk to Dr. McRae tomorrow and see what he says. You'd better try to sleep now; it's already ten o'clock."

"OK. I talked with God today. He said he might even take me to heaven tonight," she said, a soft smile lighting up her face. *"So you may not see me anymore. Good night, darling."*

"Good night, my love. God bless you." I left quickly so she would not see my tears.

"What's really wrong, Dr. McRae?" I asked the next day.

"Well, let's just call it a psychotic depression for now, because we're not sure. Her almost constant hallucinations, her hearing and talking to voices by 'ad lib' as she says, and her confused state of mind all tell us there is a psychotic disturbance going on. She definitely has a mental illness of some sort but we won't know the cause of it or how to treat it until we get all the test results. I'm booking her for a CT scan just to rule out the possibility of a tumor."

Eloper! Psychosis! Mental illness! The words terrified me.

Chapter 3: The Unforgettable Ride

Kaija did not elope again.

"You'll have to have someone sit with Kaija," the head nurse informed me the next day. She's still very restless and we're afraid she'll try to elope again. We just don't have enough staff ..."

"I know. You already told me that. But do I have to have someone here the entire day, every day?"

"I'm afraid so. She's just too unpredictable. We can handle the nights because we give her Ativan at eight o'clock and she sleeps right through until morning."

"OK. I'm not sure I can find enough people to do that, but I guess I'll have to try."

I felt hopeless and anxious. Who could I ask? I'm an independent sort and not used to asking for help. Since we've had no kids of our own, Kaija and I have learned to handle our problems by ourselves. Nevertheless, I was now forced to do something, so I called my sister, Janice.

"I need some help, Janice. I need to find someone to

sit with Kaija every day so she won't run away from the hospital again. Can you help out, and can you maybe round up some others who wouldn't mind filling in for a day now and then? It would have to be from about 9:00 AM till 4:30 PM. I can cover the evenings and the weekend."

"Of course. I'll come in tomorrow, but in the meanwhile I'll call some others. Don't you worry about it; just let me look after this. I'm sure I can get a few people to take turns."

"They don't have to be right in the room with Kaija all the time. That might get her uptight if she thinks someone is watching over her like a hawk. They can sit in the chairs in the central area near the nursing station; they can see all the exits from there. It'll make for a long day, so tell them to bring along something to pass the time. And … thanks."

Janice was true to her word. She found a different person—siblings, nieces, ladies from the congregation—to cover each day for the next two weeks. Even one of my male friends volunteered when he heard about the situation. I felt guilty, for I considered it my problem alone. Nevertheless, I was humbled and gratefully accepted the help.

It was a strange time. The hallucinations continued, but every once in a while Kaija was completely lucid. She had been for almost one whole day when her sister-in-law sat with her. But she had also become extremely angry: "What are you hanging around here for? *Do you think I don't know that you're just spying on me?* Why don't you go home—I don't need anyone here to babysit me! There's nothing wrong with me. I shouldn't even be here. But if you think I'll leave again, forget it. They don't let me go anywhere here. I'm watched like a hawk. So go home!"

"I just thought I'd keep you company," Esther replied. I had discovered that white lies were unavoidable and passed this on to the other "sitters."

Day after day dragged by. It seemed to be a waiting game. What had caused this so suddenly? Blood tests had revealed nothing. X-rays, nothing. Urinalysis, nothing. CT scan, nothing. Even the platelet count was normal at 263—nothing resembling Kaija's strange fractional numbers of 38 over 44, which sounded more like robust bust and hip measurements!

Dr. McRae called me at school, just as I was discussing Chaucer's *Wif of Bathe,* with her "hipes large" and the "remedies of love she knew perchaunce." I hoped that perchance the doctor would have some matching remedies, not for the heart, but for the mind … But I knew from Dr. McRae's first words that it wasn't going to be a simple fix.

"We've made arrangements with City Hospital to admit your wife. Since all the tests have come up negative, I think it's imperative that we get her admitted to the psychiatric ward as soon as possible so she can get the kind of professional treatment she needs. I've contacted Dr. Lowe and Emergency already. They'll examine her and arrange for probable admission. Can you get her there this afternoon?"

"Of course! I'll get someone to cover my classes. I'll be there shortly."

An hour later we were on the road, headed for the hospital in the city. I could hardly believe that this was happening. My wife! My precious wife with whom I have shared forty wonderful years! Words like "crazy," "loony," "one brick short of a load," "off her rocker," and "one cog short" echoed unbidden in my mind. I myself had used them many a time. I flushed now, in hot shame that I had done so. They'd be saying those things about my wife now.

The hour-long trip was, for me, a nightmare. Kaija seemed almost happy. She was smiling. Then she was waving gaily out her window—at nothing! Just the empty prairie!

I shuddered. Macbeth's words whirled in my mind: "Present fears are less than horrible imaginings ... and nothing is but what is not."

"Who are you waving at?"

"Just at all those people out there."

"I don't see anyone ..."

"They're over there. It looks like they're having a picnic. See, they waved back."

Suddenly it was, *"Stop! The police are behind us. They're bringing me a heart pill. Stop!"*

"There's no one behind us."

"Oh ... *Did you remember that Dad died two days ago?"*

"No."

"He did. He's in heaven now ... Dr. McRae said we're to return to the hospital right away. Listen! He's talking to you. He wants you to go with him to buy a car."

"We're not turning back now. We're halfway to the city already."

"OK ... *How much money should we send to the relatives in Helsinki and Oulu? 'Cause four more billion has come into our account. It's from the sale of Mom's book in*

China. The one she wrote about how she had to give birth to me at home."

"Come on! We don't have that kind of money!"

"We do so. I already sent two billion to the hospital foundation and four billion to the church."

Wow! That's some windfall, I thought. I chuckled inwardly, but at the same time I realized that such grandiosity was a common symptom of schizophrenia.

"Why didn't we stop before leaving town so I could see our new house that you and Lars are building?"

"We're not building any new house, hon."

"You are so. You're just in denial. You told me on 'ad lib' that the walls are all up already. But somebody wrecked them. How come you drove the truck into that slough? Will you ever get it out of there? Lucky you didn't drown. We're supposed to go to the General Hospital, you know. Elgin and Hanna are bringing me two warm blankets and a soft pillow. Will you bring me some flowers when I'm in the hospital? I should have a couple of bananas, too, to keep my potassium level up. *Don't let that guy into the car. Lock the door! He's almost caught up to us!"*

"Don't worry. He'll quit running as soon as we hit the city. We're almost there now."

"Why do we have to go to Emergency and not straight to Admissions?"

"I don't know. But that's what Dr. McRae said."

I didn't know. But I was soon to find out. This ride had seemed interminable. I hoped that ER would be less painful.

Chapter 4: ER

"Come this way, please," beckoned the nurse from behind the admitting window at ER. "We need to have your wife fill out these forms. Has she been a patient here before?"

"No. She hasn't. But I'll have to fill out the forms for her. She's ... she has a psychosis. She's not able to right now—is that OK?"

"Yes. But she'll have to sign them."

"Even if she doesn't comprehend what they're all about?"

"Well, I guess you could cosign, if you're her husband."

"I used to be, but I'm not sure whose husband I am right now. This is sure not the same girl I married." It was a lame joke, lost on the nurse, but I just couldn't get it through my head that this was my wife here beside me My earliest impressions of her when we first met flashed across my mind. Oh, yes, I had been attracted by her beauty, but beauty came a dime a dozen and I had seen and bypassed many of them. It had been a combination of her intellect and her sincerity that had impressed me. I had never talked with another woman who spoke so openly from both the mind and soul. I had never spoken to anyone to whom faith was so important and the same as my own. A sudden fear gripped me: Her mind was obviously gone—would she lose her faith as well? And would her love for me wither and die in this strange person she had become?

"Is it really necessary to fill out ALL of this information?" I asked. Do you really need her whole life history? What if I can't remember all of her previous illnesses and medications? I don't even remember the names of the ones she's on now."

I needn't have worried. As I tackled the forms with her by my side, I was amazed. She remembered everything: tonsils removed (two times!) as a youth; suffered severe pain with her monthlies for years; finally had hysterectomy when she was thirty-three years old because of deformed uterus; operated on for carpal tunnel at age twenty-two; was hit in mouth with grain auger handle and suffered concussion at age twenty-five; has had osteoarthritis most of her life; diagnosed with fibromyalgia twenty years ago; radical mastectomy because of breast cancer in 1990; and high blood pressure in 2003, followed by severe Asiatic virus and depression.

"What medications are you taking now? Can you remember them?"

"They gave me a shot of Haldol when I first went into the hospital," Kaija replied. *"It was for my blood platelets.* But it didn't do anything except make me feel confused so then Dr. McRae put me on two milligrams of Respiradol twice a day for the same thing. The first two days they gave me shots of morphine sulfate because my fibromyalgia was bothering me a lot, but it's OK now so they stopped it. They said it would help me to sleep better, too, but it just made me hyper. So then they gave me two milligrams of Ativan at night to help me sleep. I was on Effexor for my depression, but Dr. McRae took me off that when he started the Respiradol."

I was amazed. At least her memory was as awesome as it had always been. She had certainly had more than her share of health problems! Respiradol—I remembered that one because, as Dr. McRae had explained to me, "It seems that she's developed a short-term psychosis of some kind. I checked with Dr. Kardash in the city and he recommended starting her on this antipsychotic. It's the newest and best one on the market. Usually it has very positive effects within three to four months."

"What do you mean by psychosis? Is her mind gone? Is this what they call a 'nervous breakdown'?"

"Not at all. Although it came on as suddenly as what is referred to as a nervous breakdown, it's not at all the same. People who have that usually lose their short-term memory for a while and are completely helpless. She doesn't have those problems."

"So what DOES she really have then?"

"I'd call it a psychotic depression," he said. "We've been treating her for depression for about six months now, and although we seemed to have alleviated that somewhat, I'm quite sure it led to her present condition."

I felt that the doctor was trying to soften the blow for me by being deliberately vague. From the little bit I remembered from my university days, it seemed more like schizophrenia to me. In some ways it seemed similar to the classic *Dr. Jekyll and Mr. Hyde* story, yet at the same time, quite different. There were not two distinct personalities here, as in the story. Nevertheless, this seamless shifting from rational to irrational, from her usual self to this strange business of talking by "ad lib" was more than I could fathom. It blew my mind every time it happened. How was it possible?

Even with Kaija's excellent memory, it took a long time to complete all the forms. But if I thought that was a long time, I would soon find out just how short a spell it had been. After turning the forms in, we waited ... and waited ... and waited some more. The small waiting room was crowded; a steady stream of people came and went. Time dragged; there was nothing to see in the barren room, and nothing to do to pass the time. The magazines were two months old. The vending machines contained only candy and junk food. Twice in the next hour I went to the desk to ask how much longer we would have to wait. Not that I was anxious to have her admitted, but from what Dr. McRae had said, I knew that's what the outcome would be.

"It shouldn't be long now," the admitting nurse replied. "A resident doctor will be down to see her shortly. It's just been a busy night around here. Sorry."

Kaija was getting antsy. "Can't we go home already? I don't know what we're hanging around here for anyway." Three times I had to go after her as she started toward the exit. But finally we were ushered out of the public waiting room and into a private room with the usual uncomfortable hard-leather chairs. I held her hand tightly.

"Hi! I'm Dr. Anderson, a resident here at the General

Hospital. I work under Dr. Lowe, who is the psychiatrist on call tonight. How are you doing?"

"I'm just fine. And I don't need to see any psychiatrist! *My platelets are just out of whack and that's why they sent me here.*"

"Well, that may be the case, but your report shows you've been suffering from depression and indicates you've felt confused at times, so we just have to ask you some questions to be sure we're treating the right thing. Now, how old are you, Kaija?"

"I'm sixty. Or no, I turned sixty-one last fall."

"What's your middle name?"

"Lynn."

"Do you know what day of the week this is?"

"Of course. Do you think I'm stupid? It's Friday."

"And what month is it?"

"May."

"Can you count by fives for me, starting at seven?"

"Seven, twelve, seventeen, twenty-two, twenty-nine, thirty-four, thirty-seven, forty-three, forty-eight …"

"Good!"

Liar, I thought. What a big, fat white lie! Kaija's counting wasn't good at all! Why the white lie? Was he protecting her from knowing something? Was it because he himself did not know what Kaija's illness was?

"Now, can you draw me a clock face that shows the time right now?"

"Good heavens! I'm not a little kid. I did that in grade three. Anyway, *the doctor just told me I can go home.*"

"What doctor? I didn't see anyone else here."

"He told me by 'ad lib.' You heard it, too."

"Well, I actually did not hear it, and we need to

finish this examination. Please just go ahead and do what I asked, OK?"

And so she did. She drew the hands to show six fifteen. "That's PM, of course," she asserted.

For heaven's sake, I thought, and we got here at three forty-five! How long would this go on, anyway? I wanted to protest already. If I was tired, how much more must Kaija be?

"Can you tell me why you think you're here?"

"I'm here because my blood platelets are only thirty-eight over forty-four, and if they drop to thirty I'll be dead! And there's nothing wrong with my mind," she said, breaking out into tears.

"I'm sorry. I didn't mean to upset you. Here's a Kleenex … We're about done now anyway. I'll leave, but you need to stay here until Dr. Lowe comes. I'll go over my notes in the meantime and then pass them on to him. Just relax and rest—it won't be long."

So she said. Kaija's pent-up emotion and frustration reminded me of Tennessee Williams' *Cat on a Hot Tin Roof.* Every few minutes she'd get up, go out into the hall, check up and down, and then if she saw no one, make a break for the door. I had to be on my toes to catch her, and then it took some talking and a firm grip on her arm to bring her back. She'd have gotten outside once, if the burly guard hadn't barred her way. I'd have to be more vigilant, I thought, as I moved my chair closer to the door.

It was an interminable wait. Finally, at seven fifteen Dr. Lowe the psychiatrist on call, stepped in. "Hello. I'm Dr. Lowe. Dr. McRae called me earlier and told me you would be coming in. Sorry I couldn't get to see you sooner. I was with a patient. It's been a busy night!"

"I've been here since two o'clock. Can't I go home already?"

"I know you must be rather tired, but please bear with me for a little while so I can verify what the resident told me and ask you a few more questions."

Here we go again, I thought, and no sooner thought it than Kaija echoed my thoughts aloud: "Do we have to go through all this garbage again?" she asked.

"Do you know where you are now? Can you tell me what time it is now? Is this Friday or Saturday? Can you repeat the alphabet, skipping every second one? Do you remember my name? How do you feel right now? Have you ever felt that you couldn't concentrate as well as you should? Do you ever hear voices?" On and on it went.

Oh, he was gentle and kind enough, this Dr. Lowe. I didn't blame him for doing his job, but he seemed hardly cognizant of the level of distress Kaija was feeling—or me either! I was hungry, and besides it was cold in the room. I'd already given my sweater to my wife two hours ago. Nevertheless, she was still shivering.

"Have you had anything to eat? Are you hungry?" he suddenly asked.

"I'm starved, if you really want to know! We haven't eaten since noon and it's almost eight o'clock already. My hubby checked and he said there's no place to get any food here."

"That's terrible. Stay here and I'll send someone down with a sandwich and some juice for you right away." He left, closing the door behind him.

Yeah, I thought, right away in half an hour. But it

did come, in only twenty minutes. Almost as good as Domino's pizza, I thought. Yet the time was highly fraught with anxiety and therefore it felt twice as long. As soon as Dr. Lowe left the room, Kaija lay down on the cold tile floor, shoulders propped against the door and feet braced against the leather easy chair across the room. "What are you doing? Why are you lying there like that?" I asked.

"To keep those police guys out. They're scary. They tried to get in earlier when they were invisible, but I shouted at them in 'ad lib' to leave us alone." The tears rolled down her cheeks as she curled up into a ball against the door.

My poor, sweet, distressed darling, I thought, my heart aching. "Here, hon, let me move these two chairs against the door. We'll sit in them and that way no one can get in."

"I wish we could go home. *They'll be on lockdown soon.* Why do we have to stay here? I'm fine!"

Knock, knock, knock! *Wake Duncan with thy knocking, I would thou could'st,* leaped Macbeth's lament into my mind. Bring back my wife, from wherever she is, I prayed, just as fervently.

"Don't answer!" Kaija said. *"They'll kick the door down if they know we're in here."*

"It's OK, love. I think it's just someone bringing the sandwiches to us."

We ate. A half hour later Dr. Lowe reappeared. "We're going to admit you, Kaija. We need to check things out more closely and run some blood tests tomorrow. A couple of orderlies will be down in a few minutes to take you to your room. Mr. Koivu, you can go out and bring your car around to the staff parking lot to the south of the hospital. You can enter the Elliston Wing from there and see your wife after she's settled in. We'll run some tests in the morning, and you can come to see her after one o'clock." He went out and Kaija kicked the door shut behind him.

And so this chapter in our life closed with a slam. The short, yet very, very long experience in ER rated as a whole chapter, too—a very bad one. The trauma we had both gone through over the past six hours was equally as significant as many other chapters in our lives together: as significant as my career change from farmer to teacher after we had married; as significant as our move, later, from the city to an acreage so I could dabble in farming again; just as significant as our move for a few years to Arizona in an effort to alleviate Kaija's arthritic pain; and even more significant than both her breast cancer and my heart attack in more recent years.

As I got into my car to drive over to the psych wing, I sobbed uncontrollably. It was a long time before I was able to go inside. I was an emotional wreck and afraid, but little did I envision what the next chapter would bring.

Chapter 5: The Dungeon

You must be Mr. Koivu, am I right?" asked the nurse. "We've been waiting for you. Did you have trouble finding the staff parking lot?"

"A bit," I lied. I wasn't going to tell her that I'd sat for fifteen minutes in my car, trying to come to grips with my emotions.

"We've just gotten your wife into her room and settled in for the night. We had to give her some Ativan, a mild tranquilizer, because she was so agitated. She was worried that you had disappeared somewhere and had abandoned her. Follow me. I'll take you to her room and you can see her for a few minutes before you leave for home. It'll help to calm her down, too."

I followed her down the stairs of the Elliston Wing and through the dimly lit, narrow hallway of the lower level of the ward for psychiatric patients. She opened the steel door with her key. It clanged shut behind me—another door clanging shut!

I was appalled. My wife locked up? And in this hole

where the narrow windows were at ground level and barred? This was lockdown, for sure, in every sense of the word. Where had Kaija gotten that term from in her earlier hallucinations? I wondered. It must have had a different connotation for her—a drastic measure taken to counteract some outside danger, I figured. But this lockdown was for real! My own Kaija was locked inside this dungeon! Locked in with others who seemed to be locked into inner minds more volatile, or more remote, than Kaija's by far. Lockdown, as real and tangible as it was here, became a metaphor to me for that which had occurred in Kaija's mind. I couldn't access her thoughts, her inner mind, anymore; I was locked out. Nor could Kaija escape from the irrational world of fantasy or hallucination into which she had been thrown. Whatever kind of locks they were, they were strong.

"Do you expect my wife to get better in here?" I asked angrily. "This place looks like Charles Dicken's Bedlam itself!"

"Yes, I know," the nurse acknowledged." But," she hastened to add, "the government has finally approved a brand new, state of the art psychiatric hospital and it will be built next year. It's been a long time coming. This was to be a temporary ward because we've been short of space, but we've been here for three years now. I know it's not great, but it's all we have at present. And we'll do our best to take care of your wife."

"It's not only the place that bothers me," I said. "How is she supposed to get well amongst all these others who obviously are in far worse condition than she is?" I was shaken by what I saw and heard: a youngish man with his wrists taped; a young, hollow-eyed girl leaning against a door jamb; an older woman emitting a constant "aiee, aiee, aiee" as she rocked her body back and forth on the couch in the center of the small, octagonal room.

"How come she's locked up in here?" I asked in alarm. "She's no harm to anybody."

"Your wife is listed as an eloper on the forms. The doctor told us to place her here so that she wouldn't try to leave. It's standard procedure. This door is always locked. No one can get out except by asking one of the nurses on duty for permission. But you can come and visit your wife whenever you wish between 9:00 AM and 8:00 PM. Just ask one of the nurses, through the side of the office window here, to let you in. You'll have to identify yourself, of course."

Locked in! First by her own mind, and now this!

In one of the off-shaped, barren and dull rooms I found Kaija curled up under the covers in her bed. She looked lost and afraid. "Hi, hon," I said, trying to sound normal.

"How come you're here?" she asked. *"I thought you had become invisible."*

"I wanted to see how you were before I leave. I'm going to stay in town at Cindy's so I can come to see you every day. Are you OK? You look so tired!"

"I am. But you'd better go so you can get some sleep, too. *This place will be in lockdown soon so you'd better go now while you can still get out.* Good night, love," she said, giving me a kiss and a hug. She seemed distracted by my presence, as though I was intruding and shouldn't be there. So I left, and suddenly I felt all alone. Tears of self-pity flooded my eyes, but I managed to wipe them dry, realizing that if I felt alone, how terribly alone she must feel. Or did she? Regardless, this was about her, and not me, I realized. I felt guilty and ashamed.

I'm lucky to have a cousin living here in the city, I thought. It would be costly to have to stay in a motel. Cindy was shocked, of course, when I related the day's events. But she welcomed me and showed me the extra bedroom in the basement. I was glad it was downstairs where I would be alone.

In spite of the quiet and the late hour, I could not get to sleep. My mind just refused to shut down and the confusion of thoughts that whirled about in it was enough to drive me crazy! It was then that the thought came to me that I should start keeping a diary of all that had occurred since this whole bizarre thing had started. Maybe by writing I could free my mind from its jumble of thoughts and at the same time keep a record of whatever unknowns the immediate future would bring. I found a sheet of loose leaf in my cousin's computer desk and began to record the day's events.

Friday, June 3
The unthinkable has occurred: Kaija is in a psychiatric ward! Locked in, yet to boot! Of all the things I've ever thought might happen as we age, this was the very last! In fact, it had never even entered my mind. I'm afraid, because I know nothing about this kind of thing. What caused it? Will it go over quickly and she'll return to her former self? Will it change her permanently? Life suddenly seems so unreal. I feel like I'm in limbo, thrust out into space, into darkness. I am no longer in control of my life; maybe I never was, yet I always felt that I was. But if God is in control, why would he let a thing like this happen?

Saturday, June 4
Went to the hospital at 10:00 AM. Eight rooms off the octagonal common room that one enters through the locked door. Twelve feet across, cluttered with a couch, ragged easy chairs, and a small table, smack in the middle of the room. Have to walk around them to get to Kaija's room. Patients lounging about, watching the blaring TV, muttering to themselves, or just roaming aimlessly around. Sad scene!

Kaija was glad to see me. "You came!" she said. "*I thought they'd never let you in because of the lockdown. I'm surprised the police let you through the cordon. But they're gone now, so why don't you just go out and I'll follow you because I can't get out on my own—they keep this door locked all the time! We can just leave my bag of clothes here so no one will notice.*" She looked as though she hadn't slept a wink.

Sunday, June 5
Called the nurse. She said Kaija had been agitated earlier but settled down and even smiled a bit when she talked to her. She questioned her meds and wondered why she was there "with these strange people." The nurse asked me to not come for a few days so Kaija would settle into a routine. "They always do after a few days," she said. So I will not go up in the evenings after school this week

Monday, June 6
At home, now, and teaching every day. Called. Different nurse. Said Kaija is not sleeping at night. Very withdrawn. They'll give her some sleep meds tonight.

Tuesday, June 7
Talked to Kaija on the phone. Asked if I was OK. Here she is worrying about me! Didn't even ask if I was coming up. Talked real quiet; could hardly hear her.

Mind Gone Astray

Wednesday, June 8
Kills me to have to stay away. Nurse asked me to give it a couple more days. They'd given her some Seraltine, or Sertraline or something, to help her sleep. Referred to it as Zoloft also—confusing. Maybe one is a brand name and the other is generic. New psychiatrist is going to take over, a Dr. Lewis. Nurse assured me that this guy had recently received his Doctorate degree and was right up on all the latest developments in psychiatry and antipsychotic medications.

Thursday, June 9
Got to talk on the phone with Dr. Lewis. He continued the Respiradol but added another one right away—Zyprexa. Said it's faster acting, and one of the three new "second generation" drugs on the market. Too early to expect any change. Said they would be doing some blood work tomorrow.

Monday, June 13
Was home for the weekend. Took two days off school so went to the hospital at one o'clock. Doctor had given her a 10-mg injection of Acuphase, a major tranquilizer, since she still isn't sleeping. Good heavens, that's the third sleeping potion they've tried! Seemed kinda dizzy and weak. Very confused and full of hallucinations. "*Dad's gone to heaven*" was the first thing she told me. Then the conversation went something like this:

"How come you're here on Saturday? I thought you said you were going home for the weekend."

"I did. It's Monday today."

"*Oh. I was going to start walking to the River Valley church. I think I could make it to Riverview today if I walk fast. It might take me three days.*"

"Come on, hon, you can't do that! It's seventy-five miles from here. And what would you go there for anyway? You've never even been inside that church!"

"*I have to go there so the priestess can bless me. I'll have to genuflect.*"

"You're not a Catholic. And that's a Lutheran church. What ..."

"It's because they put me in here because of my sins. Anyway, the church is somewhere about Fourth Avenue and Twenty-first Street."

"That's right here in the city. I'm worried about you, hon. You're confused ..."

"I'm just fine; there's nothing wrong with my mind," she yelled, emphasis on the last word.

Friday, June 17
Didn't go to hospital for three days. Taught classes as usual. Sometimes it seems easier to not go, but then I feel guilty. They had done an ECG on her today. Not sure what that is; will have to ask Dr. Lewis.

"How come you're here at this time?" she asked as soon as I walked in.

"Why not? It's 7:00 PM."

"It is not. It's 9:00 PM. The clocks in here are all wrong. You can see for yourself how dark and dingy it is in here. You're just in denial as usual!" Projection again. She's told me that so many times already.

Poor kid. So confused. She'd written a strange note to me: *"Please call Dora as soon as possible. 306-887-3543. She wants the green thing from the middle of the flower arrangement you brought me. She said Dr. Fleuter would look after it."* Never heard of Dr. Fleuter, nor had Dora called or been there either, since she lives in Idaho!

Man, oh man, another new drug—Clopixol depot. Or maybe it's just the other name for Acuphase, since they inject it. Sounds like a bus station! Nurse says depot means intramuscular injection. Why can't they just call it that? Started yesterday by Dr. Lewis. Off Respiradol, still on Zyprexa. Can't stop right away, have to "titrate" it down over a number of days, which they have apparently been doing. What's wrong with "reducing gradually"? So much gobbledygook! Anyway, it's supposed to be for treatment of schizophrenia, amongst other things.

Visited a couple of times, but same old, same old: more hallucinations than rational moments. Can't begin to remember them all. All I know is that I couldn't invent or imagine such things as she comes up with. I guess truth is stranger than fiction after all.

Monday, June 20
Huh! Saw Dr. Lewis today and he says Kaija is not diagnosed as schizophrenic. Rather, he says, she just has a temporary psychotic disorder brought on by something. He still doesn't know what.

Kaija was allowed to go upstairs into the common area for a while yesterday. Nice and bright there. It's also where the patients from the two upstairs pods eat. These are bright and cheery, too; I hope they'll move Kaija up here soon. Another valuable feature is the fenced-in courtyard with picnic tables, a grassy area with lawn chairs, and a small garden planted by some of the patients. She said it was so nice to get out into the sunshine for a change. Was quite lucid.

Tuesday, June 21
Greeted with a very happy smile today! I cried with joy. She said she has no tears left in her. A good visit. Many signs of improvement: was doing a crossword when I got there, had sponged bathed, was interested in *The Riverview Herald* I brought, was relaxed and happy. She wanted to go upstairs and out into the courtyard, so I got permission from the nurse on duty and we did, for forty-five minutes after supper. She seemed dreamy and happy out there, but told me that *"Eileen, the school secretary, called on 'ad lib' and said you don't have to teach next week so you can stay in the city. You heard her yourself."*

When I said I didn't talk on 'ad lib' and had to teach, she gave me the old reply, *"You're in denial."* Still doesn't admit or acknowledge that she has any mental problem. Actually, I think she has repressed it and therefore is truly not conscious of her condition. However, I read on the Internet that almost fifty percent of those living with schizophrenia have no insight into their condition. Perhaps she's one of these.

Wednesday, June 22
Fair visit but I was mentally and emotionally shot so did not stay long. Kaija was quite bright, but had packed up all her belongings, ready to go home. *"You don't even love me. You don't want me at home,"* she yelled when I said she couldn't go yet today because the doctor was waiting for the results of the ECG.

Her bright moments were interspersed with hallucinations, many repeats of earlier ones but a couple of new ones: *"There's Boyd Cameron,"* she pointed out. *"He's one of the patients in here. That's my niece's boy—you've never met him. He's got some kind of mental illness. They say he's bipolar,"* and *"I need to get to a cobbler to have him make prostheses for my hammertoes and then make new shoes to fit my feet."* Never even heard of hammertoes. Asked her what they were and she showed me how three of her toes were higher at the joint and had a downward bend in them.

Saturday, June 25
Long visit this afternoon. Very rational during whole visit. I picked up two grande bolds from Starbucks in the main hospital foyer and we went for a walk by the river—first time they've let her go outside of locked quarters. Was sunny and warm. We sat on a bench in a little treed-in nook beside the bicycle path, in silence, just sipping our coffees. Private and peaceful. Kaija just gazed across the river with a contented look and was happy to just sit there in the sun and not say anything.

Sunday, June 26
What a roller-coaster ride! Today she was not herself at all and was full of hallucinations. We walked along the riverside bicycle path twice, but stayed only fifteen minutes each time—seemed anxious to get back *"because it's safer in there."* Smoking more now, five to six cigarettes a day. Says she feels better when she smokes. Took her twelve roses.

She liked them.

Our hearts break, once again, as so often happens at parting. She asks me to forgive her *"for my misdemeanor in faith."* What she means, I don't know, but I bless her anyway. As I leave the room I look back through the tiny window in her door. She's sitting on the bed weeping, so I go back in and we mingle tears once more. Then we try to give each other brave smiles, and part.

Monday, June 27
Off school for three days. Staff is very understanding. Kaija very irritable when I went today. "I can't find my cigarettes and the nurse won't let me go upstairs. This place is getting to me. I can't even see the sun! And it's impossible to find any peace and quiet in here."

Doubt if she'd leave the hospital grounds even if she was upstairs and not locked in. She's too insecure and wouldn't know where to go anyway. Met with Dr. Lewis in the afternoon. Last Thursday he started her on Seroquel, "the last of the latest generation of antipsychotics." Said they are giving her 20 mg, the maximum dose. However, he may push it a bit higher because blood tests showed that she's what they call a "high metabolizer," which means that the liver breaks down her intake very rapidly and therefore the drugs don't stay in her body long enough to be properly effective. What next!

Thursday, June 30
Last day of classes! Report cards and general cleanup. Great to be freed of this responsibility, under the circumstances. Called. Nothing new. Kaija has been pretty quiet all day.

Sunday, July 2
Kaija was moved upstairs today! We went into the courtyard and sat on the grass for half an hour and had the first decent conversation we've had since this all began. Do I dare to take these as signs that she is improving?

Monday, July 3
Took Kaija out for a haircut. She was very subdued. Stayed for supper and went outside after for a smoke. She was very tormented for the whole hour we sat there. *"There are so many rules in here that it's just like living in the Old Testament times. You're told when to get ready for bed—at six o'clock. Then you're supposed to meditate for two hours. Then you have to have some juice and a cookie at eight o'clock. Then they bring around the pills and they make you take them. Then it's lights out at nine o'clock and you can't even go to the bathroom after that."*

"Are you sure of all those rules?" I asked. "The nurses told me you'd have a lot more freedom up here."

"Yes, I'm sure. And you can't even help me because I'm in unbelief and so are you and so is all the family. That's why I'm in here and will never get out because God is punishing me for my sins."

Tried to console her and told her that this was just not true. Reminded her that the Holy Spirit still dwelled within her—even in here. She just became very quiet and did not reply a word. It seemed to reach her, though, and with teary eyes she said I'd better go because it was almost bedtime.

We parted in tears, but not before preaching the gospel of forgiveness to one another, the nucleus of our faith. It was comforting, the only comforting moment of the whole long day.

Tuesday, July 4
Dr. Lewis met with us at nine o'clock. Kaija was very defensive and it was obvious she still has no awareness that she has any mental problems. When Dr. Lewis asked if she knew why she was in the hospital, she said, *"For my depression and my blood platelets."* Then he asked if she still heard voices, to which she replied angrily, *"I don't hear voices! But people talk to me all the time on 'ad lib' and they warn me when there are bomb threats. God talks to me sometimes, too."*

Not sure if this is a hallucination or a delusion, this ability to talk directly with God. But so much for my hopes of improvement. Dr. Lewis said that if the meds don't soon work, they could consider ECT (electroconvulsive therapy), but only as a last resort. Said he'd have to get Kaija's and my OK to do so. Sounds ominous to me.

Friday, July 7
The date of our engagement. Got a nice surprise to celebrate it, too. Dr. Lewis came by in the morning and suggested I take Kaija home for a three-day pass! Of course I agreed, but I also expressed my anxiety about how this would go. He said it would be good to see how she reacted in her home environment and that way he could have a better reading on how she was responding to the Seroquel. My heart soared.

So, after the meds are ordered, we'll head for home this afternoon—together!

Chapter 6: Roller-Coaster Ride

I picked Kaija up at 2:00 PM. She was sitting outside at the picnic table, tears in her eyes. *"I thought you had died,"* she said. I assured her that all was fine and that we could go home now. That elicited a big smile, and after picking up her pills from the front desk, we walked out the door and into the sunny afternoon. Before leaving the city we stopped and got a double chocolate ice cream cone and strolled through the park by the river, enjoying it. She didn't have much to say, but her face held a soft, happy look. I hoped the entire pass would go this well.

The drive home sobered me. Hallucinations I had not heard for a long time came tumbling out: *"Are we going to our new house now? It's so sad that most of the family is in unbelief. They'll all go to hell. I can't greet you with 'God's Peace' as we always do because I'm not believing either. Do you think Dr. Naipaul will be waiting for us at the new house? He's better now."* There were plenty of new ones, too: *"I'm going to sell 2500 round bales of hay to Marvin for a dollar each. They're bringing us a new dresser today. Ron and Carol's baby drowned in a water puddle on the street yesterday. Carol's family has already gone down there."* Was it just the sudden release into freedom that had also released all these hallucinations? I wished I could understand this illness better. Maybe at home in familiar surroundings she'd be herself.

We drove straight to the hairdresser's since I had made an appointment for her to get her hair cut. The shop was full of people. We had to wait twenty minutes, and Kaija was so antsy I had a hard time keeping her there. Either she didn't like being among so many people, or the rather loud hum of the air conditioner above our heads bothered her, for five times she got up to leave. I had to block her exit and quietly encourage her to wait just a bit longer each time. The haircut itself went OK, but it was a silent one. Before, she and her hairdresser had always chatted up a storm.

At home, Kaija was so full of hallucinations that evening that I didn't even try to record them in my diary. I was too exhausted and depressed. The next morning was no better. She woke me at six o'clock and wanted to go to *"the new house because the others are already there."* She could not find her glasses so she put mine on. When I said they were mine, she merely gave them to me and continued on downstairs, no concern about where her own were, or even if she had any. Downstairs she began to pour a *"big cup of coffee for Gary Thornton because he's upstairs fixing the computer. It just starts building files for no reason."*

At 8:00 AM she packed up her bags to go somewhere—likely to the new house. There was a jumble of stuff in them that she had dug out of her dresser drawers and the closet. She would have taken her morning pills again if I hadn't caught her. She didn't remember me giving them to her earlier. The most disconcerting moment was when she walked out the door while I was on the phone. When she didn't come back in after a few minutes, I cut the call short and went out. I couldn't see her anywhere. I panicked. I jumped into the car and drove down the street. As I turned the first corner, I saw her standing at the next street corner, gazing at a relatively new, white bungalow across the street. Likely she was wondering if this was our "new house."

"Why did you leave and go walking down here on your own?" I asked angrily. Maybe it was more fear than anger, but in any case I then said the wrong thing: "You're having hallucinations or something."

"That's a lie! Don't you ever say that again!" she shouted vehemently.

At lunch she was totally within her newly created world. I picked up my sandwich. Kaija's lips moved silently as she communed with someone. What was she saying? Who was talking with her? Occasionally she'd smile. She would look right at me. I'd smile at her, but she didn't see me at all. To me she said not a word. It was as though I was invisible. After lunch we went out for a smoke, and on the front lawn she began waving at *"Larry McEcheran. He works at the town office, you know."* There was no one in sight.

In the afternoon she was again tormented by voices telling her that she was not believing, that no one in the family was, and that she wasn't, either. I talked to her gently, telling her not to believe those people on "ad lib" because they always lied. I blessed her and assured her that she was still in faith. After a few minutes of silent contemplation she said, with a beatific smile on her face, *"I've repented."* Nevertheless, the rest of the afternoon she was mostly mute and staring and would do nothing but lie on her bed. I tried to draw her out by chatting with her and then by playing her favorite Mary Beth Carlson CD, but she seemed to find this irritating and asked me to turn it off. No doubt it distracted her from the conversations going on in her mind.

The evening was worse than ever. She was in tears much of the time, talking to her voices, sometimes angrily. I could see that she was a tormented soul. I, too, was tormented, just to see her this way. How much heartache must I suffer? I could bear it no longer so I took her back to the hospital that same evening. She went without a word of protest.

I felt like a tattletale as I related to Dr. Lewis, who fortunately was on call, why I had brought Kaija back early. She had been vacant, staring, silent during the entire drive to the city. She had walked into the Elliston Wing very slowly, dejected, depressed. Nevertheless, when I went to her room, she appeared relaxed and almost content.

"It's late, and I need to get to bed right away, so you'd better go" was all she said. I decided to not even go to see her on Sunday; it seemed that she didn't really want me there.

We both met with Dr. Lewis on Monday morning.

"We're going to change the antidepressant medication from Zoloft to Desipramine," he told us, "as we can measure the amount of this drug in the system more accurately and thus tell how long it stays in the body."

"OK," I said, even though I hadn't realized that she had been on Zoloft. I thought she had been on Effexor the whole time.

Dr. Lewis then explained that he would start giving Kaija twenty-five-milligram Clopixol injections, starting immediately, and continuing every two weeks. This way, apparently, the medication would bypass the liver and stay in her system longer.

"We often treat fast metabolizers this way, Kaija, and you are one of these. I'm confident that this will have positive results after three or four injections. The other thing we could try, as I mentioned before, is ECT."

Kaija was adamantly against it *"I won't take any electrical treatment! I don't think it's even right! You just want to give me a frontal lobotomy!"*

"No, we won't do that. Yes, there are some minor risks, but don't you think it's worth a try to see if it would get rid of those voices that plague you so much?"

"They're not voices! They're real people! I talk with them all the time. God talks to me, too."

That ended that discussion. My mind was awhirl with doubts and questions. Were any of these neuroleptic drugs doing any good? Some of them, according to Dr. Lewis' own admission, could cause disastrous side effects. I recalled how McMurphy, in Ken Kesey's *One Flew Over the Cuckoo's Nest,* became an experiment as Nurse Ratched attempted to metamorphose him from a rebellious to a catatonic state. And what about this ECT business? With McMurphy the shock treatments were disastrous. Kaija had read the novel, too, just as she had read all of the novels I studied in college. Was that where she had gotten the idea that ECT would lead to a frontal lobotomy, which was McMurphy's eventual fate? How ironic life could be! *Cuckoo's Nest* had been one of my favorite novels of study. These questions of the mind, which had so intrigued me then in fictional form, were now a regular part of my life! I surely knew now that truth could be stranger than fiction. As bizarre as McMurphy's experiences had been, I felt that my own experiences with Kaija were, to me at least, even more baffling.

The next day Kaija was much better as we walked along the bike path by the river. She spoke hardly at all, but she held my hand and seemed content. The following day as we were out on a drive she asked, "Why did you bring me back here anyway?"

"Because you were so unhappy at home and having so many hallucinations ..."

"I never had any hallucinations! Name me one hallucination I had!" So I told her some of them. She just listened. No response. Neither admission nor denial.

The rest of the week went better. We did something together every day just to get away from the psych wing for a while. One day we went on a picnic lunch in Riverside Park, another day to tour the aboriginal museum, another just for her favorite praline ice cream and a Starbucks coffee. Still, she was far from normal and I was somewhat surprised when Dr. Gates, who was taking Dr. Lewis' patients while he was on vacation, arranged for another three-day home pass. But maybe it will go better this time, I thought.

It was, and it wasn't. We went to RJ's for lunch with her brother and his wife, and Kaija was fine. The next day we went to her sister and husband's for a visit and sauna.

She wasn't very talkative, but what conversation she did have was normal.

But in between the good times were segments that were very, very bad. The first evening Kaija had been wild with hallucinations: *"Dr. Naipaul is back in the hospital ... we should go to our new house ... Mason is eloping tonight ... Laestadius and Luther and God are all on live 'ad lib' ... Luther is criticizing my clothes—he says I should wear bloomers instead of panties ... my sisters and brother are all smoking again ... Linda's husband went back to Jamaica and married another woman ... John, the nurse today, is invisible ... "* and on and on.

The next morning as Kaija came downstairs it was, *"They told me that you were gone and that I'd have to go back to the hospital and stay there for three years!"* Then at breakfast she complained that *"these voices even tell me what to eat and what not to eat,"* and then blurted, *"Randall, stop using dirty words!"* The next day had gone OK, but I noticed that she had a lot of short-term memory loss, not recalling, for example, that we had gone for groceries and later for an ice cream.

On Sunday, the third day, she had again been tormented by extremely negative hallucinations on the drive home from her sister's: *"They're going to drop bombs tonight and the whole town will be on lockdown ... Take me to the funeral home—Dad died and his funeral is tomorrow ... "* and on and on again. I didn't know how to respond and just replied with "Oh" or "I see." Then she started on again about Dr. Naipaul and the new house, that Dr. Naipaul was going to live there with us, that the furniture was going to be delivered tomorrow, etc. I had gone head-to-head with her on this, refuting her every assertion, but to no avail. When I told her she was hallucinating again, she shouted as before, "There's nothing wrong with me!" I doubted that I was handling her right, yet I felt that I had to get these bizarre ideas out of her head somehow or she'd never get better.

On Monday morning I had a major struggle getting Kaija to return to the hospital. It seemed as though life was beginning to be a series of concentric circles, the common center being my struggles to get Kaija back into treatment after each failed trial to have her at home.

"I won't go back there! *There's nothing wrong with me except that my platelets are sticking,*" she shouted.

"You've told me that a hundred times already," I shouted in return. "But the doctors have yet to confirm anything about that. In fact, the blood test results are right here. You've seen them yourself …"

"Those aren't mine, I've told you! They're someone else's …"

"Why can't you believe what the doctors tell you, for a change? You've gotten to be so stubborn …"

"Shut up!" Kaija shouted, and crawled back into bed.

Four times I tried logic and reason, and four times I was stonewalled. I finally resorted to trickery. I packed up her things, put them in the car, and appealed to Kaija to "go see the doctor just so we can get some meds for your platelets, and then come back home." She reluctantly agreed. I breathed a sigh of relief; at least this time I would not have to use physical force, something I had feared might eventually happen.

We arrived at the hospital at noon, but had to wait until two thirty to see Dr. Lewis. While waiting, I had to talk her into staying put a half dozen times, and even had to physically restrain her twice. Then, when meeting with Dr. Lewis, she asked him, "When did Charles talk to you? That's why I have to stay, isn't it? Well, I won't stay!" she shouted, and bolted from the room.

She was right about that; I had talked confidentially to Dr. Lewis, but her own behavior condemned her, too, and Dr. Lewis ordered that she be placed in the "Dungeon" again. My guilt cut into me like a knife in the heart. I had never felt so badly. It was my fault that she was in the Dungeon again!

This collaborative coercion hit me even harder when, the next morning, I was handed an official document: "CERTIFICATE OF MEDICAL PRACTITIONER FOR COMPULSORY ADMISSION TO AN INPATIENT'S FACILITY." The word "compulsory" confirmed my feeling that I had been an accessory in sending my wife to prison.

The form outlined the practitioner's general reasons for this action:

(a) Said person is suffering from a mental disorder and needs treatment and care or supervision that can be provided only in an inpatient facility; (b) as a result of the mental disorder, the said person is unable to fully understand and make an informed decision regarding his/her need for treatment and supervision; and (c) as a result of the mental disorder, the said person may cause harm to himself/herself or suffer substantial mental or physical deterioration if he/she is not detained in an inpatient facility.

In spite of my guilt, as I read through the fine print, I had to admit that, on the basis of the three points, she did need to be in the hospital to receive the kind of care that would hopefully make her better, and that I could not give her at home. It gave me some consolation. There were two identical forms, in fact, each one annotated and signed by a different examining psychiatrist.

As I read their notes, my sense of consolation soon waned. Dr. Lewis' report reiterated what I had already been told: Kaija had "psychotic depression … no insight into her illness … needs hospital management of meds and ECT."

The second examining psychiatrist's notes were in greater detail, but the highlights were that "Mrs. Koivu has widely fluctuating moods; her affect was blunted; she reacted very angrily when her beliefs regarding her direct communication with God were discussed, reflecting the extent to which she still holds her delusions. Her insight remains limited."

Even though I already knew all this, I wept. To see it in writing gave it such a sense of finality, of doom.

Chapter 7: ECT

This readmission was a scary one, for I suspected that Dr. Lewis would want to start the Electro Convulsive Therapy treatments, and I was right. He had gotten another opinion from Dr. Gates, he explained, and they wanted to start them right away.

"It's nothing to be afraid of," he assured us. "We attach electrodes to the side of your head, near the temples. The electrical pulses are carefully controlled, and they're not strong. They're nothing like what you read about in horror novels or see in the movies such as *One Flew Over the Cuckoo's Nest*, where the person's arms and legs twitch and often the whole body convulses. That's all fiction. The pulses or shocks are so mild that there is practically no physical response at all. We have had a high success rate with these treatments and we feel that since the medications have not worked, we should give this a try."

Kaija listened in silence, and began to show signs of acquiescence by asking, "How long does it take?"

"It takes from twenty to thirty minutes each time."

"That's such a long time," she complained. "Will I have to be under an anesthetic?"

"Yes, of course. You won't feel a thing. We'll give you from eight to twelve treatments, one every second day. Usually eight treatments are sufficient."

I wasn't so sure that the treatments were as benign as Dr. Lewis had made them sound. The Wikipedia entry read: "When the general anesthesia has taken full effect, the patient's brain is stimulated, using electrodes placed at precise locations on the patient's head, with a brief controlled series of electrical pulses. This stimulus causes a seizure or convulsion within the brain, which usually lasts for approximately a minute. Side effects may include headaches, muscle soreness, nausea, confusion, and partial loss of memory for the days, weeks, and months preceding ECT."

It was the words "seizure" and "convulsion" that made me shudder. However, as I read on I was somewhat reassured and my guilt over my part in the whole situation was somewhat lessened. "ECT will produce a substantial improvement in at least 80 percent of patients. (Surely she'd be one of this 80 percent, I thought.) It is no more dangerous than minor surgery under general anesthesia, and for some patients may be less dangerous than treatment with medications. Researchers have found no evidence that ECT damages the brain. The seizures occur under controlled conditions and MRI scans verify that there are no changes in brain anatomy. The amount of electricity that actually enters the brain is much lower in intensity and shorter in duration than that which would be necessary to damage brain tissue."

"That many treatments means I could be in here for a whole month" was Kaija's immediate reaction.

I knew how she felt. I felt so sorry for her; she had already spent nine weeks in the hospital!

"Will she still be on the medications?" I asked.

"Yes, but we're taking her off Desipramine, the antidepressant, during this time, but will continue with the Seroquel and the Acuphase."

"What's that, actually?" I asked.

"It's another neuroleptic. That's what antipsychotic drugs are called. Actually she's had it before, just under another name. It's similar to the Clopixol shots she's been getting. She's due for another one tonight."

Here we go again, I thought. I was thoroughly confused by all these names. Why did they have to have so many different names for all these medications? I had tried to keep on top of things by looking up on the Internet every one that she had been on, but the wealth of information and the variety of drugs seemed endless.

"We need to meet, though, with a social worker and any members of your family you'd like to be present to make a final decision. Could we meet tomorrow afternoon?"

"Of course! I'll call Kaija's brother and sister to come. I'd feel more comfortable if they were here, too."

But Kaija's seeming acquiescence was just that—a seeming one only. Her brother and sister—and I, too, for that matter—felt that the treatments should be tried. But all throughout the meeting, no matter what anyone said, Kaija was adamantly against it.

"I won't take the treatments, no matter what you say.

Just take me home," she repeated angrily and defiantly, over and over.

Dr. Lewis then explained that since the family wanted her to have the treatments, and since Kaija was against them, they would have to have an appeal hearing with himself, two other psychiatrists, a lawyer to represent Kaija, Kaija herself, and me present. Other family members were welcome, too. This was done so that treatment that was deemed necessary under extreme circumstances such as this could be given even against the patient's own will.

Once again there were two copies of an official form: CERTIFICATE FOR ELECTRONCONVULSIVE THERAPY. Why did they have to use such a negative word as "convulsive?" I wondered. I shuddered again. Again there were the general reasons: (a) The patient's mental condition will improve significantly if ECT is administered; (b) alternative treatments have proven to be relatively ineffective for treating the patient's disorder; and (c) the patient's mental condition will not show significant improvement without ECT.

Déjà vu, déjà vu, I thought. Around and around we go. Once again there were the opinions of two examining psychiatrists. "I have formed this opinion on the following grounds: eight weeks of trials with two atypicals, one typical, two antidepressants, supranormal dose, with no meaningful improvement to psychotic depression. APA Guidelines have ECT as first line of treatment for psychotic depression." These were Dr. Lewis's detailed comments. Dr. Gates, the other psychiatrist wrote, "Mrs. Koivu has shown only limited improvement from various antipsychotic medications that have been tried. It is important to continue the course, and she cannot give informed consent.

I did not see any reason for Kaija's sister and brother to be there. They had expressed their opinion already, so I told them that I could handle it alone.

"You will be given every opportunity to express your feelings at the meeting, Kaija. The lawyer is there to help you, to see that your rights are honored, and to ensure that you get a proper hearing. After the hearing, the doctors and the social worker will meet and a ruling will be given on whether to go ahead with the ECT treatments or not."

That afternoon was hard on me. Kaija repeatedly begged me to take her home. As evening came on, she became desperate, clutching at all sorts of straws: *"They'll be on lockdown tomorrow and you won't even get to the meeting ... World War II is starting tomorrow! I'd have to die here alone ... Don't keep me here! If you don't take me tonight, I'll get Clare to take me for a walk in the morning and then I'll start walking home."*

Hard on me? I felt ashamed at even thinking about myself when my loved one was in such torment and fear. But was there really any other choice at this point? It seemed that they had tried every new neuroleptic, and a couple of older ones, too, and all with no results—or very short-lived ones. Before I left in the evening, I asked the nurse in charge of Kaija if she would give her a whirlpool bath to help relax her and then a sedative for the night. She promised to do so.

The appeal hearing decision came back the next morning: "Your appeal has been DENIED in accordance the requirements of The Mental Health Services Act."

"We'll start the treatments this afternoon," said Dr. Lewis. "The anesthesiologist will come by and get your medical history in an hour or two. Don't be afraid. I'll be there to see that all goes well."

Kaija seemed resigned to the inevitable. She answered the anesthesiologist's routine health questions directly and clearly, and was in turn reassured that the medical team cared about her and that all would be fine.

I went to the hospital early so that I'd be there when she was brought back to her room. I was surprised. I wasn't sure what I had been expecting, but Kaija looked perfectly fine. She even smiled.

"How are you, hon?"

"I'm fine," she said, with an almost contented sigh. "Now that's done." She obviously thought that it was all over, forgetting that there would be many more treatments.

"Now I can go home!" she said.

It was hard, hard, for me to say it, but it had to be done. "No, darling, you can't go home now. Remember what Dr. Lewis said? They have to give you at least eight treatments for them to have an effect."

This provoked a litany of desperate attempts to convince me otherwise: *"The administrator said I could go home right away. If we don't go home now I'll have to stay here forever! You hear the voices, too—they're all saying I can go home now."*

Kaija was almost frantic. Three times she went to the door to see that she wasn't locked in. She wasn't, but a male nurse barred her way each time. Twice she went to the front desk to beg the nurses to let her go. Finally, as I just watched in dismay, she packed her belongings into a plastic bag, set them outside her room, and told me, matter-of-factly, "I'm ready to go."

I wept. Kaija comforted me. Role reversal again, I thought. I kissed her good night and left, my heart torn in two. Once again, I felt like a schmo.

Chapter 8: Passages Home

If I thought I had been jerked around emotionally to this point, I was soon to learn that there was to be a frenetic series of uppers and downers that made the previous roller coaster ride seem like a kid's ride, indeed. Whether there was a shortage of hospital beds, or nurses, whether the psychiatrists were overextended, or whether Dr. Lewis believed that Kaija would benefit from intermittent passes home, I never did learn. More than likely the repetitive pattern that was to emerge was due to all of these factors.

I had no quarrel with the doctors or the nurses. On the contrary, I was very pleased with Dr. Lewis' tenacity in trying to find a treatment and medications that would lead to Kaija's recovery. And I couldn't fault any of Kaija's many nurses in the Elliston Wing of the City Hospital. They were understanding and compassionate. In spite of being overworked, they meticulously and daily charted Kaija's responses to the various treatments. Another factor, for which I was really grateful, was that they had time for me—time to explain Kaija's every behavior, reaction, hallucination, emotional ups and downs, and above all, any slight improvement or signs of recovery. They helped to keep hope alive in me.

Nevertheless, I was not prepared for the strain that would be put on my hopes over the next few months. I never knew what to expect as each new home pass occurred. Everything seemed so tentative, so unknown, so experimental.

Those first two passes, fraught with hallucinations, had shaken my confidence that she would soon recover. I felt so helpless, but I was willing to do anything that might be beneficial to my loved one. At least when she was home I was able to observe and try to understand her swings in emotion and behavior myself, and perhaps—just perhaps—I could draw her out of her inner mind and have some influence on her recovery. I was determined to be as diligent as the nurses in tracking Kaija's improvements and, if it so happened, her regressions as well.

Pass Three

Driving home from the city, I was pleasantly surprised at Kaija's interest in her surroundings and by the animation in her voice. She sounded like a bird set free, like Maya Angelou in *I Know Why the Caged Bird Sings*. Simple, commonplace things attracted her attention: "Did you hear that meadowlark? It seems there's one on every second fence post ... Looks like the harvest will start pretty soon since the wheat is turning so much already ... There sure are a lot of hay bales in the ditches."

"I'm so glad to see you so happy, hon," I said. "Are you glad to be getting home?"

"Yes," she answered simply, a glowing smile on her face.

As we drove up to our home, the conversation took a little different twist: *"Why are we coming here? I thought we were going to the new house. Dr. Naipaul is waiting for us."*

"Hon, we don't have a new house. This is where we live. Let's go in, OK?"

She didn't argue. As she walked into the kitchen, she looked around, smiling, and commented, "You sure keep the place clean. You're still my same good hubby."

"I cleaned things up just for you, my love. I wanted things to look nice and I didn't want you to have to be cleaning on Saturday." I drew her to me and let the warmth of her body flow into me. "Should I start to make supper already?"

"You don't have to do it. I'll make it. *I wish I could cook as good as Jerry Gorman, though. He made such good soups at the hospital.* Did you ever meet him, or was that before we started going together?"

"No, I never met him. He was in your brother's grade in high school, you told me once, and that was long before I met you."

"Oh. Well, I'll fry up these pork chops you took out. Shall I do them in Golden Mushroom soup?"

"Sure. We both like that." And so she made supper, or most of it. I had to help her with the mashed potatoes, though, because "I don't know how much milk and butter to add," she said, confusion in her voice.

On Saturday she made porridge for breakfast, salmon

sandwiches for lunch, and cooked up some chicken breasts for supper, all on her own. I could hardly contain my joy in seeing her back to her normal self. As we ate supper, though, I noticed that she would disappear into her own thoughts and sometimes she would be mouthing words, obviously in conversation with some inner voices. But the hallucinations seemed to be benign, at least, and did not last long. After supper we went for a drive and then spent the evening reading. Kaija spent a long time looking through a new cookbook I had bought, with just this thought in mind that she might be interested enough in it to draw her out of her inner self for a while. It worked, and I felt good. Such a little thing, yet it was the first time I felt that I was able to help her in some way.

"You make breakfast this morning, OK?" she said the next morning. *"I never work on Sundays but it's OK for you because you're a man. Just make some toast, though, because the nurse just told me I'm not supposed to eat much today because of my blood platelets. Our new house is ready now, so after breakfast we'll go over there. They're going to bring the new jackets from your school to our new place. All the students have signed them."*

"None of those things are true, hon! I wish you wouldn't listen to those people on 'ad lib'; they always tell lies."

She was silent. I wasn't sure if I should refute her when she expressed her hallucinations, but I figured that if I could help her understand that these inner voices were not real, maybe she would start to accept her condition and by doing so, begin healing. I expected her to argue and say, as usual, that I was "in denial" but she didn't.

Nor did she get angry, as she usually did when I talked about her voices. This wasn't so bad, I thought. Kaija's hallucinations were more benign and definitely fewer than the last two times. I could handle a few hallucinations.

The day went well. Kaija enjoyed visiting with a number of people after church, and we spent a fun afternoon chatting and reminiscing at my sister's. My sister and her husband had been married just a few months before Kaija and me so we had a lot in common, only they had had a large family while Kaija and I had not been able to have children at all. Sometimes, now, I wish we had, for I wouldn't have felt so alone in my struggles. But I really had no regrets; I had married for love, not children, and my love for her was stronger now than ever before.

I felt reluctant about taking her back to the hospital, but I knew I must. Although the weekend had mostly gone well, there had been those few times ... and now, when the moment of truth arrived, I knew that I had let my hopes soar too high.

"I don't have to go back. There's no bed for me there ... the place is full ... they've changed the certification ... I don't need any more treatments."

She had an answer ready each time I said that we had to get back before 8:00 PM. I felt sorry for her, for I would not have wanted to leave my home and go back there either. Finally, I had to phone the Elliston Wing and talk to the nurse while Kaija listened. When she heard the nurse say that they were waiting for her to come back, she grudgingly accepted the fact. "OK," she said, and got ready to go.

The trip back was uneventful, but the silence, *the silence of the lambs,* was deafening.

* * *

Kaija was given her third ECT treatment the next morning.

"I feel better this time." Kaija smiled as she was wheeled back into her room. "I guess I'm getting used to it."

"You look better too, my love. I'm so happy to see you smiling!"

"You brought me some saffron carnations! They're so cheery! Thank you!"

"Shall I get us a Starbucks and then, after you've rested awhile, we can go out and sip them at a picnic table?"

"You know I'd love that. Bring me a dark fudge brownie too, OK?"

Kaija was in better spirits than I had seen her for months. Could the ECT treatments actually be doing some good? Dare I hope, once again?

I stayed at Cindy's. On Tuesday Kaija was again in good spirits. At noon I went downtown to Bob's Used Books and bought four books on the royal family for her. Two of them were about Princess Diana, and I knew she would especially like them. I picked up a bagel with lox and cream cheese—her favorite—and again we enjoyed it outside.

I got myself a Caesar salad from the mall and we ate supper together. Later we again went to the mall and enjoyed a banana Frappuccino and an espresso brownie. Kaija was scheduled for a whirlpool bath at seven thirty so I left early and went back to Cindy's. I felt relaxed, and even happy. It had been a good day!

I met with the doctor on Wednesday morning. Dr. Lewis was pleased with Kaija's progress.

"She's coming along well," he said with a smile. "I'm thinking we will probably be able to release her after the eighth treatment. But it's a bit early to tell, yet."

"I sure hope so. It would be a relief if these treatments would be more effective than the antipsychotics she's been on up till now."

"Well, we'll know by the end of August …"

"I hesitate to say this because it will sound as though I'm not real keen on having her home again. But that's not the case. I'm just a bit worried because that will be just before school begins again, and I won't be able to be at home with her during the days."

"Let's wait and see. We don't have to make a decision now, but if she keeps on improving it may work out fine."

After her fourth ECT treatment that afternoon, I broke the news to her that I was going to attend my nephew James' wedding in Minnesota. She was devastated. "I've never felt so rejected in my life. I didn't think you'd go," she said. That made me feel so badly, so selfish that I almost told her that I'd not go. I didn't have to.

And yet I did. I felt I just had to get away for a bit for my own mental health. The nurses, the doctor, and the social worker that I had spoken with yesterday about Kaija's possible release had all been pressuring me to take a break. Apparently the strain was showing on me, and they all repeated the same litany: "You've got to take care of your own health, too. How can you help your wife if you're not healthy yourself?" I had been disgusted at the suggestions at first. After all, it was Kaija's health that was at stake! But gradually I had begun to see that they were probably right, and so I decided to take a five-day break and go to this wedding. I arranged for Kaija'a brother, Lars, and his wife, Lillian, to take Kaija to their home on a short pass for Saturday and Sunday.

That afternoon, I almost changed my mind again. Kaija's hallucinations abounded: *"Don Singer has died ... They're having trouble with the dam again and it's leaking ... Heavenly Father says I can't stay here ... I can't even smoke outdoors in this city anymore ... I won't have to come back here Sunday night because they've cancelled my next treatment ... You'd better phone Lars when you get back to see if I'm still there."*

Perhaps it was because she had not slept well because another patient had been screaming off and on all night that she was so out of it.

I tried to get her interested in looking at the royal family album in the evening, but she was listless and only glanced through it for five minutes. She was tired, and so I left early. It was a sad, sad parting, harder on me than on her because of the guilt I felt for abandoning her for five days. I forced myself out the door and into my car. The dark rainy night did nothing for my mood.

Pass Four

I called Kaija from Minnesota on Friday. The ECT treatment had apparently gone well, but she sounded flat and tired. Some friends from the city had visited her both Thursday and Friday evening. I had arranged that, and I was glad they had been willing to go. *"Esther and*

Walter (her sister and brother) *would have come too, but they were locked out,"* she said to me on the phone. *"How come you're down there now? You don't love me very much, do you?"* I could think of no possible response to such an accusation.

I called Lillian on Monday evening when I got home from Minnesota. The pass had generally gone so-so. Kaija had had a lot of hallucinations, chief among them that the dam was going to break, so she had refused to sleep upstairs and had merely dozed on the sofa all night—in her clothes! They had awakened to her prowling around the house more than once, and once she had opened their bedroom door to see if they were there. She had told them that she did not have to go back to the hospital except for a checkup in one year. Nevertheless, when it came time to take her back Sunday evening, she had reluctantly gone.

* * *

Kaija was out of the Dungeon and back upstairs when I arrived late Tuesday morning. Although she daily expressed a wish to go home, she had shown no signs of trying to leave for the past two or three weeks.

"Your wife was telling me last night and this morning that you had died," Angie, the nurse, told me. "But she said it so matter-of-factly, and showed no signs of grief over it. She was also worried that the dam was going to break and that the city would be flooded. But she seems happier now. Her ECT treatment went well yesterday."

"Hi, hon! I'm so glad you're back. I was lonesome for you. Did your trip go OK?"

"Yes, it was all right, but I missed you so very much that a lot of the time I didn't really enjoy it. I just felt that you should have been there with me."

We spent a pleasant afternoon together. I went and got us some Kentucky Fried Chicken for supper. Kaija enjoyed that. She read the *Reader's Digest* while I read some poetry that I would soon have to teach to my grade eleven classes. We did a crossword puzzle together and she was much sharper than me, as usual, in getting the blanks filled in. In the evening before I left to go to Cindy's, I washed her hair. I asked Angie to see that she got a whirlpool bath before going to bed that night.

I had to attend a school conference the next day, but when I arrived on Thursday morning, I noticed a visible tremor in Kaija's left hand. She'd had her sixth ECT treatment on Wednesday; I wondered if the treatments were causing it. But they had recently increased her Seroquel "to full strength," too, and that may have had some effect as well.

Dr. Lewis came by later and told me that because the anesthesiologist would be away on Mondays, Kaija would have to have her next treatments on Tuesdays and Thursdays. That meant only two a week instead of three, prolonging the whole affair. I felt frustrated. Besides, we would have to attend another hearing tomorrow to get recertification for more ECT treatments, a safeguard to protect the patient, I was told. I wondered what the psychiatrists' comments would be this time. Lately I thought that Kaija seemed to be improving quite significantly, yet there were still those disturbing hallucinations.

The routine hearing was held at eight thirty Friday

morning: "Psychotic depression; demonstrating partial response early to ECT; incomplete and unsatisfactory response to several antipsychotics; still no insight into illness" were Dr. Lewis' succinct comments. Dr. Benita Lan, the other psychiatrist, had written, "Mrs. Koivu has had some improvement with ECT, though limited. It is important to continue the course and she cannot give informed consent."

I felt pretty sure the appeal would be "DENIED." It was, but perhaps out of compassion, they granted Kaija another three-day pass home.

Pass Five

Although the drive home was uneventful, when we arrived home Kaija was very flat, unhappy, even morose. She merely lay on the bed all afternoon and the hallucinations came spilling out one after another:

"We have to go to the new house right after supper ... They've mixed Maxwell House coffee in with our Edwards coffee—it's bitter ... The cheese got put into the car trunk in the city ... Sklar is going to send us boxes to ship our sofa and chair to Toronto for re-covering; they'll do it for free, just for Kaija and Charles ... The Midtown Sobeys has set aside thirty pounds of chicken breasts for us ... Cindy said she put too much garlic in the pasties ... those twelve pairs of jeans you bought me are at the other house ... There are twelve pairs of new panties at the new house, too ... I can't wait to wash clothes in our new Miele washing machine at the new house ..."

I was appalled by these, but I was struck dumb by her announcement after supper: *"You'd better get ready for your memorial service tomorrow."*

"But I'm right here, hon. I haven't died," I told her.

"But you came back. Uncle Rick has come back six times."

I had no answer to that. I left the bedroom, went down to the kitchen, and wept. In the meanwhile, Kaija packed all her notions, jewelry, and clothes into plastic grocery bags *"to take to the new house tomorrow."* After she had fallen asleep, I quietly unpacked them.

After a ten-hour sleep she seemed refreshed and lucid on Saturday morning. She didn't even notice that I had unpacked her bags. I made dinner, and as we ate, it began again:

"I talked to Toby (our dog that died five years ago) *last night ... Dad's funeral is at 3:00 PM today ... The Sklar furniture needs to be sent tomorrow, and we'll have it back in three days ... Martin will be down to 160 pounds this fall; he's 220 now ... We should go to the new house to get my new clothes; Dr. Naipaul, Craig and Renee, the whole family are all there now ... "*

And once again I felt that I had been hit between the eyes when she asked, *"Did you go down for a viewing of your body today? Are you going to your wake tonight?"*

I lost my patience. "No, I didn't! And there's no wake, since I'm not dead!" I replied in utter frustration and dismay. "Look, I'm right here at the table with you. How can I do those things when I'm not dead?" Kaija just looked at me and didn't say a word.

That afternoon I had to remind her many times that we were going to be going to her niece's wedding at 5:00 PM. She lay on the bed, talking silently *"to Esther."* She wouldn't tell me what the conversation was about, but it went on for a long time. When it ended, she seemed to notice me suddenly and it began again:

"The wedding has been moved to another town; we don't have to go. The guy at the powerhouse at the dam said I should not wear white to the wedding because it would distract from the bride's gown ... James and Miki are both going to work at the mine way up in Cigar Lake ... The post office is holding twelve bottles of Fleur de Rocaille cologne for me ... Carlo and Vivian are leaving for Finland tomorrow; they're going to stay there for three years ... Where's that ugly, heavy coat the school gave you?"

Kaija was fine during the wedding ceremony but visited only halfheartedly with the other wedding guests at the reception. Afterward, she appeared very tired, confused about the day and the time, and went to bed early. I was worn out, too, and we both slept a ten-hour night.

I hoped Sunday would be better, but Kaija had a dazed look and complained of a sore back. I felt somewhat dazed myself after these last two days, but she soon began to put me through the wringer again:

"City Hospital has sent more meds to Riverview—you'd better go pick them up ... Linda is at the new house waiting for us. She came with the new Ikea car that Alfred bought for her ... They're shipping our Sklar furniture tomorrow ... Toby says she liked to curl up on our Sklar furniture when we had it in our other house ... Belinda asked us to come for dinner, but we can't go because she's at work ... Let's go to the new house to see the new coat you bought me and my new bread-making machine ... Dr. Naipaul is waiting there for us to come for dinner ... We have to go to the post office at seven thirty tomorrow morning to have our picture taken.

They'll take a picture of us sitting on our Sklar furniture—it's all for advertising ... Dr. McRae and Dr. Lewis just said I should not be on Seroquel ... "

I didn't try to refute any of her claims. There was no point. I could see that her hallucinations were as real to her as reality itself. In the evening, as I sat in the La-Z-Boy trying to read, I could hear her talking aloud to herself upstairs. I tried to ignore it, but discovered that I couldn't remember a thing about the last ten pages I had just read. When I went upstairs to suggest she get ready for bed and go to sleep, she obeyed me like a little puppy and soon drifted off into a peaceful sleep.

I was pleasantly surprised at her response the next morning when I told her we had to go back to the hospital. Actually, she was not due back until eight that evening, but I felt sick about her state of mind and wanted her to get back under professional care as soon as possible. Besides, I didn't think I could get through another day like the last three had been.

She gave no resistance. "I'm sure this will be my last week," she said. I hoped so, too, but I had heavy doubts.

* * *

The stay in the hospital—a short one this time, from Tuesday to Thursday only—passed uneventfully. I was glad, because I was back teaching school now and couldn't be up in the city to see Kaija every day.

Her eighth ECT had gone fine, according to the nurse, when I called Tuesday evening. Dr. Lewis called me on Wednesday at school.

"Although we had positive results from the first few

ECT treatments, Mr. Koivu, it appears that this early improvement has leveled off. Therefore, I want to give Kaija another four treatments. However, I need Kaija's and your permission for this."

"I'm not very happy about these treatments," I responded. "It appears to me that the tremor in the hands is becoming worse as these treatments go on …"

"That's true," the doctor interrupted, "it has increased lately, but the cause is not the ECT treatments. It's the residual effect from the Seroquel we've had her on. It's unfortunate, but it's a side effect patients sometimes have to that particular neuroleptic, and we can't reverse it. Later on, we can try to lessen it with Propanolol; right now, however, we have other, more important issues to treat."

"I don't consider it a minor issue, though. It means that she can't crochet, or even read or write anymore because of the tremors. These have been her hobbies in the past, and now she's deprived of these ways to stimulate her and to pass her time."

"I understand, Mr. Koivu. But let's concentrate on the main problem just now—eliminating the psychosis that is controlling her life."

"Yes," I agreed, "but do you really think further treatment will help?"

"I think so. But I need to know if you'd be in favor of temporal lobal ECT treatments. The only difference is that we'd attach the electrodes nearer Kaija's temples instead of high on the forehead as before. This sometimes has a more direct effect on the targeted areas of the brain. It's just as safe, and it's a sound procedure that we do often.

"I suppose so. It sounds scary to me, but I can only trust in your judgment. And since the treatments so far have produced only minor improvements, I guess it's worth giving this a try."

"If we have to, we can still continue the Clozaril depots. These can easily be administered by home care nurses, too."

Was that a hint that Dr. Lewis was confident that these last ECT treatments would produce results and that Kaija would soon be able to come home? "OK, I'll talk with Kaija about it this evening."

When I phoned Kaija that evening, she was quiet, subdued, and I noticed a trace of fear in her voice. "What's wrong, hon? You sound afraid."

"They're going to operate and give me a frontal lobotomy," she whispered.

No wonder she was afraid. "No, love. That's not what they're going to do. Dr. Lewis asked if they could do a temporal lobal ECT. That's not a brain operation. They're not going to operate and remove anything. You've confused it with a frontal lobotomy, which is such an operation. All they are going to do is place the electrodes in a different area, more on the side of your head instead of on your forehead. Otherwise all will be the same."

"Oh. Then I suppose that's OK. This will be my ninth ECT. I thought Dr. Lewis said eight would be enough."

"He did think so, originally, but he's not satisfied with the progress, so he wants to try four more, this way. Let's try and look on the bright side and keep our fingers crossed that these will work better. Esther and Walter will pick you up tomorrow shortly after your morning treatment and bring you home. I should be home from school by four thirty. I love you."

Pass Six

When I arrived home from school on Thursday, Kaija was delighted to see me. She thought that I had become invisible again since I was not there when she arrived home with Esther and Walter. But she heated the homemade beef stew that I had taken out of the freezer in the morning, and supper went just fine.

In the evening I had her type up a couple of pages of school documents for me. Although she still had a tremor in her left hand, she was nevertheless better coordinated and focused than she had been the last time she did this, two weeks ago.

She was OK at home alone on Friday while I was teaching. I phoned her twice just to make sure she was doing all right. But as I arrived home, I no sooner got in the door than she said, *"Dr. Naipaul is waiting for us at the new house."* I pretended I didn't hear and quickly changed the subject. From there on the evening went fine, but a new hallucination popped up just before bedtime: *"Arlene* (the landlady of our duplex) *has gone away. We have to watch because people could squeeze between the bars of the back gate and then squeeze in under the door. If so, we're supposed to call the police."* I assured her that I would watch, and she fell peacefully asleep.

Saturday morning Kaija was absorbed in looking through old scrapbooks in our cedar chest. At lunch she was bright and happy; the memories of the past had obviously stimulated her. But the landlady was still on her mind: *"Arlene is going to sell the house and we have to move to our new house. Dr. Naipaul will help us unload. Are there boxes in the basement so I can start packing?"* I told her there were no boxes, and she dropped the issue immediately.

Later, in the evening, the same issues resurfaced: *"Dr. Naipaul has been waiting for us for an hour already ... Turn your cell phone on—Arlene is trying to call you to see when we're moving."*

Then, out of the blue she announced: "I got this virus from a boy in China."

It was the first time she had alluded to the possibility that this may have been at the root of her illness. I had often wondered about this myself, for certainly it was during our last two months of teaching ESL in China for two years that her blood pressure had risen, her weight had begun to drop sharply, and the doctors had not been able to find any cause. It had been the reason for our earlier-than-planned return to Canada.

A new behavior pattern developed that evening as she was getting ready for bed. She shut the lights off in the bathroom and locked the door, *"because anyone on 'ad lib' can see me and watch."* Poor girl, I thought. She didn't need such paranoia on top of everything else!

Kaija's fibromyalgia bothered her all day Sunday so she basically remained in bed. I sat up beside her, reading, but was often interrupted: *"We need to stop at Dr. Naipaul's on our way home from church ... That boy in China gave me that virus I had ... They're sending more meds out from the city ... Make sure you double lock the doors tonight. Donovan, the security guard, will watch over our place. He'll bang once, loud, on the door if he wants in."* I replied in monosyllables and this appeased her. I was thankful that at least her hallucinations weren't the tormenting type this time.

Monday, Labor Day, was not a good day. The hallucinations about Dr. Naipaul and the supposed new house were repeated at least three times, but this time with the added twist that we were going to celebrate her sixtieth birthday there. The biggest problem arose when I told her I had to take her back to the hospital because she was still having hallucinations. That was a mistake, I realized, for it made her extremely angry and forced her into denial.

"That's not true. I don't have any hallucinations. There's nothing wrong with me except my blood platelets. You just don't want me home. It's your fault that I have to go back. Well, I'm not going!"

Would I ever learn how to relate to her when she was like this? I wondered. I did my best to keep my cool, but it was extremely difficult for me to convince her that we had to go. She kept getting various "ad lib" messages, each with a different reason she did not have to return. Twice I had to phone Brenda, the nurse in charge of her, while Kaija listened, to verify that they were waiting for her to come in before eight o'clock. She was extremely upset with me and blamed me for it.

When I finally got her to the hospital, she tried one more plea: *"Dr. Delbert* (the premier of the province), *just said I can stay at home."*

It was another hard parting for both of us. Kaija wept deeply. *"I feel so rejected! You made me come here because you don't want me at home."* After a while, I was able to calm her down and we blessed one another before we parted.

* * *

Tuesday and Thursday Kaija had her tenth and eleventh ECT treatments. When I called her Tuesday evening she wept on the phone. She wanted to come home so badly. When I talked with the nurse Wednesday evening, she told me that Kaija had tried to leave the building several times.

On Thursday afternoon, Esther and Walter again brought her home for the weekend. I wondered about this in-and-out of the hospital pattern. Yes, I wanted her home, but in the state she had been in lately I felt she would be more stable if she did not come home so often. It seemed to just upset her when she was not allowed to, or able to, follow up on the messages from "ad lib." Her blaming me each time did nothing for my mental health, either. However, I had no option but to rely upon the doctor's opinions and wisdom.

Pass Seven

"Oh, there you are," Kaija said, as she met me at the door after school. *"They told me that all day you were feeling poorly because of a blood clot in your heart."*

There on the table, packed into plastic grocery bags all ready to go to the "new house," were her notions and some clothes, a few bananas, and both my and her medications. Beside them were her purse and a thermos of coffee. After gently but persistently explaining to her that we had no new house, she sadly began to unpack and put everything back into its place. I went into the bathroom and wept bitterly. Such a sad homecoming!

Things didn't get any better. The rest of the day she

was full of hallucinations: *"A lady phoned me and gave me Dr. McRae's home phone number ... The pharmacist has some blood pressure pills for me that you have to pick up at seven thirty ... One of your students is in my ward now—she's bulimic ... I don't understand why your sister has it in for me ... Edgar and Hannah left a carton of cigarettes for me ... The minister from Finland said I've smoked over my quota today. He stands in for the heavenly Father sometimes."*

Friday was no better. Kaija went on and on about the furniture at the "new house," the new clothes that I had supposedly bought her, the fact that "everyone" was waiting for us at the "new house," until I was so frustrated that I had to get out and go for a walk.

On Saturday Kaija was very demanding: *"Go pick up my meds from the drugstore ... Alorie is sick and in the hospital. Get over there right away—they're waiting for you ... We need to get to the new house right away ... Dr. Naipaul is waiting for us at the new house, let's go already."*

Since I could not comply with such demands, I tried a new tactic—I'd change the subject, and this distracted her. It felt like an epiphany, this discovery of how to deal with her. It sounded so crass to put it that way. I had never had to "deal with her" before. Ours had been an open and loving relationship, but as things were now, I found myself floundering so often, unsure of how to relate to her. It frustrated me, but most of all, it left me bewildered and sad.

Amazingly, Sunday went well, with hardly any hallucinations. We went to church, and later to a wedding reception for James and Miki. Kaija was absorbed the whole afternoon reading through their old love letters that I had dug out of the trunk for her.

I was somewhat afraid to leave her at home alone on Monday when I went to school, but I wanted to try it again to see how she would make out. I had taken out some soup for her to warm up at noon so she would not have to tackle what for her had become an almost impossible task—first deciding what to eat, and then knowing how to go about making it. At noon I got a call from Esther, telling me that Kaija had called and told her that I was very ill and in the hospital. I called her right away and reassured her that I was at school and was feeling fine.

I asked her about this when I got home: "Why did you think I was in the hospital, love? Do you feel better now that you see me here and that I'm not sick?"

"I know you're here," she said, somewhat annoyed, "*but your other self has already come back and is sick and in Riverview Hospital.*"

I had my hardest struggle yet in trying to get her to go back to the hospital that evening. Kaija simply refused outright, went upstairs and into bed, covers pulled up tight. I talked and talked, gently at first, then firmly, all to no avail. Finally, in anger, I tried to physically lift her out of the bed—not a good tactic, I knew, but my patience had reached its limit. Seeing my determination she compromised, saying that if we phoned the hospital and the doctor wanted her back, she would go. I phoned. She listened. Reluctantly she got into the car.

As we drove toward the city, I came to realize why she had been so very reluctant to go: *"They're going to do a frontal lobotomy on me,"* she kept repeating. I felt like a rat. No wonder she had resisted me so strongly this time! If only I had known her state of mind earlier ... but then, would it have changed anything?

* * *

Kaija received her twelfth ECT on Tuesday. On Wednesday I got a call at school from Dr. Lewis. "We're going to stop the ECT treatments. She's plateaued, just as she has on each of the medications we've tried. We'll let her recover from the treatments, so you can take her home until next Monday. We'll start Clozaril shots then next week. But first we'll run an EEG and a SPEC scan. Tomorrow we'll have to have another hearing to extend her hospital stay another ten days or so because we'll want to monitor the effects of the drug. Maybe after that she can be released to Riverview Hospital and Dr. McRae can do the ongoing blood testing that's necessary."

"This will be the eighth time we've tried a home pass," I pointed out in exasperation. "It seems like we're going around in circles and getting nowhere. Sure, I'd like her at home, but this coming and going is really upsetting, to both Kaija and me."

"I know. But we can't keep her in hospital indefinitely ..."

Pass Eight
The hearing on Thursday morning was routine, with the usual reasons the psychiatrists felt she should be held in the hospital for further treatment, even against her will. Kaija's appeal to be released was, of course DENIED. As we drove home, I had to agree with the decision, for

she was anxious and full of hallucinations. I was glad I had decided to take the next two days off school.

"The roads will be real icy the last fifteen miles," she said as soon as we left the city. *"There's lots of snow in Riverview. They just said the snow is wet and heavy and the snowplows are getting stuck."*

"It's still only mid-September, hon. There's no ice or snow yet, so don't be worried," I reassured her. At home Kaija was no better. Just before bedtime she announced, *"Why are we eating supper here instead of at the new house? ... Ben and Shirley and Barry and Mabel are coming over to visit us there after supper."*

I told her it was too late for company and headed upstairs to get ready for bed. Kaija did not follow me right away so I went downstairs to see why she hadn't come. Here she had made two full thermoses of coffee and dug some bars out of the deep freeze for the company! After she went upstairs, I dumped the coffee down the sink.

Friday was uneventful, yet the hallucinations continued: *"Donovan, the guard, was here. I left a big black mug of coffee on the table for him ... We can smoke in the basement now. Arlene said it was OK because she's going to paint anyway ... Diane said for me to come early for a haircut because she has to leave for home early ... You need to go pick up my pills from the pharmacy sometime today."*

While I did some schoolwork on Saturday, Kaija washed a couple of loads of clothes. She appeared to know what she was about, which I was pleased to see. She did not wash the bed sheets, though, *"since we're moving to the new house."* Other than that, she had a relatively good day, resting for most of it, but looking through old scrapbooks off and on.

Her birthday would be on Monday, so on Sunday after church all of my brother's and sister's families came over, bringing birthday cake with them. Kaija was delighted, yet she had little to add to the conversation. Later she informed me that *"they're having a birthday celebration for me at the church in the evening."* That, of course, did not occur, but in the evening her own brother and sister and their spouses came over with another birthday cake. Again, she was pleased but very subdued, wholly unlike her normal self when she was with her family. I noticed that the shake in her hand was worse.

The pass ended on Monday as all the others had, with a struggle to get her to return. But I was used to that now and so it did not bother me as much as before. I had learned to accept what I could not change, and Kaija's natural desire to be at home was one that I neither could not change nor wanted to change. I wanted her home, and it was hard for me to have to take her back, against her will, each time. With each pass I had dared to hope that she would have improved; with each pass I had to admit that she had not. It had been a frustrating few weeks with the intermittent passes, each one bringing her no closer to a permanent stay at home. Would the circle ever be broken?

It seemed cruel for me to admit it, but now, after the fact, I would rather have had them keep Kaija in the hospital the entire time. Nothing had been gained by the passes, and this jerking us about so frequently had taken its toll on both of us. At least in the Elliston Wing she had been under constant observation, monitoring, and treatment, and had become used to the daily routine. That was one of the important things I had learned from my reading: Routine is necessary for those with psychosis. It reduces their anxiety, helps them to feel comfortable and secure, and thus enables them to better think and heal. I could not even begin to imagine how hard these forced returns to the Elliston Wing must have been for her. They had been hard on me, too, but that was a minor issue compared to what my honey must have gone through.

Chapter 9: Home Again!

Instead of keeping Kaija in the hospital in the city for another ten days as had been planned, Dr. Lewis released her to the Riverview Hospital, "because Dr. McRae can do the blood tests to monitor the Clozaril medication, and she'll be happier to be close to home."

I wondered about that. It seemed as though they were trying to get rid of her, pass her off to someone else. Did they just need more beds in the Elliston Wing? Or was it that her latest six-week stay had long since passed and even though it should have been obvious to them that Kaija had only slightly improved, they were anxious to get her out of the Elliston Wing? I had learned that six weeks was the longest they could keep a patient against her will; to continue to hold her meant going through the formalities of an appeal hearing again. Did they really feel that Kaija had improved enough to be released from a psychiatric ward to a normal hospital? How could they assume that she'd be happier in Riverview? She might just as easily feel even more frustrated at being just a few blocks from home, yet not allowed to go there. It had been from Riverview Hospital that she had eloped in the beginning—what if that pattern reasserted itself?

Of course Kaija was delighted when I picked her up at five thirty. She was going "home"—at least she knew she was going to Riverview. Her nurse, at my request, wrote a short note explaining very clearly that they were transferring her to Riverview Hospital so she could be among family and friends. I wondered if Kaija really comprehended that, but to my amazement, she entered Riverview Hospital willingly and settled in just fine.

The hospital stay lasted a week. She did not have to have someone stay with her as she did the first time, for she was no longer considered an eloper. However, because I wouldn't—or actually, couldn't—take her home, she cried and cried the first night when I went to stay with her after school. She told me I was *"in denial, as usual."* Thereafter, almost every evening, she had some "logical" reason she should be released: *"I can go home now. Dr. McRae wrote a release this morning already ... I can go home tonight because they're having a birthday celebration for me at seven o'clock ... They're having a fortieth anniversary celebration for us at the church tomorrow so I can go home tonight."* I noticed that the tremor in her left hand was worse again.

According to the nurses, the first few days Kaija was flat, then agitated in turn, sometimes keeping to herself and talking in whispers to her voices, at other times roaming the halls, waiting for me to come and take her home. But as the week wore on, she brightened up. She smiled and talked rationally when I was with her in the evenings. I'd usually bring her some treat: a cappuccino, a praline ice cream cone, a small, bright bouquet of fresh flowers. Not that there weren't hallucinations, but they were not nearly as rampant as before. The blood tests revealed that her blood count and calcium levels had remained normal.

On Friday Kaija got another pass, but this time an open-ended one. She could come home to stay, as long as all went well! That last phrase was the clincher, but I was willing to gamble on it; it had been over five months since the beginning of the psychosis. It seemed much, much longer than that, so it was only natural that I longed to have her home again, hopefully to stay. I prayed it would be so.

Kaija was ecstatic; I was somewhat less so. I knew full well that she wasn't cured, for I remembered the doctors' warnings that one was never fully cured of such a psychosis, but could only reach various "degrees of recovery." I thought I was psychologically ready to accept that now, especially since Kaija had been much better these last few days. What were a few hallucinations, after all? I had learned, albeit the hard way, to counter and to cope with these. They certainly would not change my love for her; in fact, I felt I loved her more now than ever before. Perhaps it was a protective instinct that made me feel this way. It didn't matter. What mattered was what I felt in my heart, and there I felt only hope and an overwhelming relief that she was back home.

My relief was short lived. The next four weeks were fraught with both old and new hallucinations, but these didn't bother me so much. It was a number of new developments that got to me as time wore on. She packed boxes and suitcases for moving to our "new home" almost every second day; she was extremely reluctant to go anywhere with me, and often would not go; she talked loudly and vehemently to her voices; she began to dress and undress in a darkened, locked bathroom; she was tormented by people "poking at her leg." Most frustrating and disturbing, she fought against taking her meds and going for further medical tests.

The packing issue came up the Sunday after Kaija came home. I tried to get her to go to church, but she refused, saying, *"I can't go. I have to start packing all this stuff so we can move to the new house."* On Monday it was a repeat of the same words. Both times I managed to talk her out of it, but on Tuesday when I got home from school, I found that she had carried cardboard boxes up from the basement and packed up everything in our bedroom! She was angry with me when I began to unpack it all, but she eventually pitched in and helped me, berating me the whole time for being in denial.

When I came home from school the next day, I found that she had removed the electric can opener from the wall and packed it, the toaster, coffee pot, and thermoses in a box. *"This place is sold, so we have to move,"* Kaija said. Pork chops I had set out for supper she had put back into the freezer, *"because we'll be eating at the new house."*

Two days later I came home to find Kaija dressed up in her Sunday best, the rest of the clothes in her closet set aside on hangers ready to go *"to Dr. Naipaul's. Esther and Walter, Lars and Lillian, and Darla and Henry, all of my family, are there at the new house for supper. I need to get new shoes, but you told me in the morning that we can go tomorrow, so I'll just wear these ones tonight."* She made no attempt to start supper *"because we're going to Naipaul's,"* so I had to fry the fish and boil the potatoes myself.

I noticed that if I did not refute her but rather distracted her by going on doing things as normal, she would often forget her hallucinations. But it was wearing on me, this constant issue about packing and moving, and having to unpack things all the time.

Five times on one Saturday Kaija urged me to get boxes and begin packing. Twice when we went visiting, she cut the visit short by putting on her coat and stating, *"we have to get home already so we can start packing."* Another day, when I phoned her from school, she told me she was busy packing. Sure enough, when I got home, I saw that she had dragged the two largest, black Air Canada suitcases up from the basement and had them packed full. I lost my temper that time, and unpacked in a fury as she lay on the bed, just watching me, submissive and subdued. I took the empty suitcases out to the car and locked them in the trunk.

Twice more Kaija hauled empty boxes up from the basement, these times into the living room, and packed them full of ornaments. I should have gotten rid of the boxes, too, I reflected. But then, she would likely just have used plastic shopping bags, as she had done in the past. As I looked back over my notes of the past month, I counted nineteen times that the packing issue had come to the fore. That was more than every second day. No wonder it was getting on my nerves!

What got to me most was her newly acquired tendency to talk, sometimes quietly, but more often loudly and vehemently to various voices on "ad lib" that seemed to be tormenting her. Some evenings, as she lay on her bed, there was an almost steady stream of conversation. At one moment, she would be smiling and talking in a sweet and quiet voice, the next she would be angrily ordering people to leave her alone. I could hear it as I prepared my school lessons in my office across the hall, and it would distract me so much that I would often have to move downstairs to work at the kitchen table.

One night at the supper table I could see that she was listening intently to her voices. She then took a sticky note and wrote: *"Fasting blood sample Friday at 7:15 AM."*

"Are you ready?" she then asked.

"For what?"

"They said they're waiting for you."

"Who?"

"The family."

"What for?"

"To have a meeting."

"About what? I don't know about any meeting."

"Don't talk like that. You heard them. There's something wrong with you, too."

She was right about that. I had never felt so stressed out in my life. I had, in fact, made an appointment for myself to see a different psychiatrist than Dr. Lewis, to see what I could learn about handling the frustrations and the anxiety that had been gnawing at me lately. I was constantly on edge—maybe the psychiatrist could teach me how to keep my cool and cope with the situation. Or perhaps he could prescribe some kind of medication that would level out my mood swings and decrease the anxiety.

Soon the talking to the voices began right away in the morning: *"Don't touch me! Leave me alone! You don't know anything and besides it's none of your business!"* It continued off and on throughout the day and became an evening ritual. Kaija would go into the bathroom to get ready for bed, lock the door, and shut the lights off as she had done earlier. Then the whole time she was "sponge bathing," as she called it, with antibacterial Wet Ones and brushing her teeth, she erupted into loud talking: *"Leave me alone! Stop it! Get out of here. You're not even supposed to be in here. I know how to brush my teeth without you nattering on about it."* Sometimes it went on for ten minutes. Often the poor tormented soul would come out in tears and I would have to quiet her down and comfort her as she crawled into bed.

A similar situation soon developed in which she was also tormented and driven to tears every time. I awoke one morning to her crying out, *"Quit poking my leg!"*

"What's going on?" I asked in consternation.

"Those people keep poking me in the leg. It wouldn't be so bad if they didn't keep jabbing at it all the time." There followed a whole string of other hallucinations, and then a repeat about her leg: *"Dana and Lars keep poking my leg! I can't stand it!"* she said in tears. I couldn't stand it either—not the talking this way, but the tears and anguish she obviously felt. It must be a true, physical pain, I thought. I wondered if her fibromyalgia was acting up and this was her way of explaining the ache it caused.

"Don't you do that again or I'll hit you," she would often say. *"I said quit that!"* When I asked her what was happening, it was invariably a variation of: *"These people keep jabbing needles into my sore knee and thigh. Lars, quit that! Leave me alone already!"* Sometimes, when she was most agitated and in obvious pain, she would switch into

Finnish, her native language: *"Heita pois! Ala koske minua! Sa olet semmoinen hevosen perse! (Quit it! Don't touch me! You are such a horse's ass!)"* She would rub her thigh, or I would often rub it for her, and eventually the pain (or was it just a somatic hallucination?) would go away, as would her tears.

It was the business with her meds that worried me the most and eventually led to the sad ending of her stay at home. The first thing Kaija did when we arrived home was to cross the Clozaril off her list of medications. Not a good sign, I thought, not knowing how prophetic a thought this would turn out to be. That night, and the next and the next, it was a regular battle to get her to take it.

"The prescription was cancelled," she would say, or, *"There's warfarin in it. I'll die from kidney failure,"* or, *"Dr. Lewis said I don't have to take it anymore because it will cause a calcium imbalance."* I tried every trick I could think of to get her to take it, but to no avail. Finally, one morning it became a shouting match as I lost my temper and imprisoned her in the kitchen until she finally, angrily, took it, with the usual retort, *"You just want me to die!"*

Of course I protested, and tried my best to reassure her of my love. Sometimes we would make up and bless one another with the forgiveness of sins. At other times she went to bed angry and I was left with an ache in my soul.

Finally, one night she absolutely refused to take the pill. She grabbed it from me and threw it down the sink. I felt sick with despair. I phoned City Hospital and asked what I should do about it, as this was one of the two antipsychotic meds she had been on since coming home. The nurse suggested just leaving it for a while and trying again an hour or so later. No deal; it didn't work. I then phoned Dr. McRae, and talked with him as Kaija listened in. The doctor talked to her a long time. Finally, he said, "OK, don't take it tonight, but come and see me at the clinic at ten o'clock tomorrow morning and we'll talk it over some more."

When we got off the phone, the excuses started again: *"That pill has been taken off the market. Millions in the USA have died from it. Five people in City Hospital died from it this week."* The upshot of the doctor's appointment the next morning was the compromise that she could be off it for ten days, and they would reexamine the situation again at the next appointment. The doctor and Kaija agreed to keep the dose of Seroquel at the same level for the time being.

Three days later, Kaija would take only 350 mg of Seroquel instead of the 450 mg she had been taking. The next day she cut it back to 300 mg and the day after to that to 100 mg. We had a couple of big fights over that, but she came out the winner. The next day she refused to take it altogether. I was beside myself. What was I to do?

Her next appointment date with Dr. McRae was in a few days, so I did nothing. Kaija's hallucinations multiplied as each day passed: *"Queen Elizabeth slapped Charles' hand with a fly swatter when he didn't eat properly ... I heard what went on between all those parents and teachers today ... We have to be out of here tomorrow because they're starting to renovate ... How can we go to the city for my shoes when there's three semitrailers jack knifed on the highway ... We don't have to go to the doctor because he's gone on holiday … Would you please butt out when I'm trying to eat … The computer's building files again so I unplugged it and the printer … I can't drink orange juice or milk, or eat eggs because there's too much calcium in them. You go and ask Dr. McRae what I can eat … It's Thursday, not Friday … Dr. Naipaul has supper ready for us … we need to go to the Esso to drain the gas tank because the car heats … my prescriptions have all been cancelled … I don't have to go for that nuclear SPEC scan; it's been cancelled."*

My heart sank. I had been afraid she wouldn't go for the scheduled test. She was adamant about it: *"Five doctors told me I don't need that test and I'm not going."* We had a regular row about it twice, but of course that accomplished nothing. And she now refused to take any of her pills!

At the appointment, Dr. McRae could not get through to her either. She was angry with him and walked out into the waiting room. Dr. McRae told me that he would fill out a Form A for involuntary admittance to the City Hospital and for me to return her there so they could get her back on medication. I felt sick inside. I knew what that meant—another major struggle.

I was right. Kaija refused to go. At a loss what to do, I called her brother, Lars, to come and try to talk to her and convince her that she needed to go. Lars tried his best to explain patiently and logically why she should go, but Kaija was beyond logic. Logic means nothing to an irrational mind. I could have told Lars that, but then, what other means was there to approach her? Kaija just became even more angry and adamant. She wouldn't budge. She made a tactical error, though. Instead of remaining in the safety of her bed, she went out onto the deck for a smoke. I followed, and locked the door behind us.

"Why did you lock that door?" Kaija screeched. "You're sure a low-down, mean shithead! I have every right to be here as much as you."

"Of course you do, but since you refuse to take your meds, you simply have to go back to the hospital so they can put you on some new ones. You're not better yet, and you need them."

"You'll have to go one way or the other," Lars said, blocking the exit stairs from the deck. "You can't stay here on the deck all night."

"I won't then! Let me past! I'll go and find my own place to live."

"You know that's not possible, hon. If you'd only stayed on your meds, this wouldn't be happening. I can't make you get better here. You need professional care right now. Please, let's get in the car and go. They're already waiting for you at the Elliston Wing. I know it's not what you want, but there's no alternative now."

"Well, I won't go. I'll sit here till I die."

I was in a quandary. What was I supposed to do? How could Lars and I get Kaija into the car without forcibly carrying her there? I wouldn't do that. She'd fight like a cornered animal and likely get injured in the process. Besides, I had never used force of any kind on my wife and I wasn't about to start now. But what should I do?

In desperation, I called the police and explained the situation, stressing that Dr. McRae had given me the required legal Form A, necessary to involuntarily admit one to the hospital. The police in turn called an ambulance. Both arrived at the same time. It looked strange to see the police car parked in front of our house, and the ambulance backed up on the driveway. It hit me hard. What a step I was taking! How drastic for me to call the police to take my wife away! The irony of the situation hit me—here I was, creating, as it seemed to me, a totally irrational and abnormal action, sending my wife away with the help of the police. How had the tables turned this way? I felt as though everything was taking place in another world. My mind was in a fog. I couldn't think.

I wondered if the police would use force to get Kaija into the police car. What was their role here, anyway? Why had I even called them? Why hadn't I just called the hospital and asked the doctor on call for advice? How could I be doing this to Kaija? Maybe I should just …

"We're only here to help you and your husband," said one of the policemen. "We came because your husband called and asked us to come. He knows he has to take you to the hospital against your will, but he's doing this only because he cares about you and wants to help you get well again."

"Yes," the second policeman chimed in. "We're not here to strong-arm you into the car and whisk you away. We're here to help you to, help you to make the right decision. And the right decision now is not to stay home but to go to the hospital. You're not well. You need doctor's care …"

"I don't need any doctor's help! All I need is to get something for my platelets. They're sticking. And the count is too low. That's why I'm weak and need to rest all the time."

Jesse, the first responder, took a cue from that. "Kaija, we've known each other a long time. You know I'm here to help you both. Even if it's only your platelets that need fixing, only a doctor can help you with that."

"They'll never let me come home again," Kaija wailed. *"They'll keep me there till I die."*

"No, dear, that just isn't true. You just need to get the doctor to get you on some different meds. Who knows, he may be able to do this right away and send you home again. But in any case, you need to see a doctor to get the help you need. Come. You won't have to go in the police car. We'll take you in the ambulance. You can just lie down comfortably and rest all the way there."

Jesse had a soothing voice and a soft, gentle mannerism. She was good with people, and good at her job. She spoke gently, yet she was firm and reassuring at the same time.

And so, Kaija went. Likely it was Jesse's soothing talk that worked. Or perhaps it was the realization at seeing the police and ambulance personnel all gathered there that she would have to go one way or another. She finally allowed Jesse to lead her into the ambulance.

"Can my husband ride in here with me?" Kaija asked, now somewhat calm and above all, compliant.

"No. But I'll sit here right beside you. We can chat while you rest. Your husband will follow us in his car, right?"

"Of course," I replied. "I'll be right behind you all the way, and then we'll go in to see the doctor together."

It was a long, long drive. I had called the police to take my wife away! How could things ever have come to this pass? How could I do such a thing, treating my wife as though she had committed a crime? You could hardly call not taking meds a criminal act! Maybe it was all my fault. Maybe I had approached her the wrong way about the importance of taking her meds. Maybe I should have been gentler—gentle yet firm, as Jesse had been. I surely shouldn't have become so frustrated and angry. This had only made Kaija even more determined not to take the pills, or the shots. I had always been short on patience; if only I had been more patient, maybe she would have complied. But what did I know about how to handle someone with a psychosis of any kind? I should have asked a social worker about that, or at least I should have done more reading on the subject. One could find any information one wanted on the Internet. Why hadn't I thought of that? I kicked myself.

And yet, was there any alternative? I could not handle, nor could I help, Kaija any longer. Things had not been good right from the start, but they had been especially trying since she had quit taking her meds. That was really the reason she had to go back. But maybe I could have managed …

The truth of the matter, however, was that no matter how I tried, I was unable to help her in any way. Although my action seemed cruel and unjust, I salved my conscience with the knowledge that I was helpless to help her, and that only professional care would get her back on track. It was already the end of October; Kaija had been at home for only twenty-seven days. The immediate future looked as dreary and bleak as the late fall day. And I still felt guilty.

Chapter 10: Back in the Dungeon

I was devastated when they put Kaija back into the Dungeon. Now I really regretted forcing her to come back to the Elliston Wing. I hadn't expected this! She was virtually a prisoner again, in an archaic facility that was hardly fit for criminals. My heart bled for my poor loved one. How could she cope with this all over again, especially after getting a taste of freedom and home? The many-hour ordeal once again in ER had been hard enough on both of us. Kaija had almost slugged a guard in her anger and agitation when he wouldn't let her leave. After that, the guard stood outside the room the whole time.

"Why in heaven's name are you putting Kaija down here again?" I asked the doctor tersely.

"We have no choice," said Dr. Lee, the psychiatrist on call. "Because she fought coming back so strongly and was delivered to us by force in an ambulance, it is standard procedure to place the patient in here. We can't run the risk of her eloping. It's not only to protect the hospital personnel from liability, but to protect her as well."

"What do you mean 'protect her'? She's not the least bit suicidal!"

"That's not what I was concerned about. We're close to a main street here with a lot of traffic, as well as to the river. It could be dangerous if she eloped in a state of anxiety and wasn't fully cognizant of what she was doing or where she was going."

"How long will she have to stay down here?"

"We can't tell that in advance. It depends on her behavior, and the availability of a bed upstairs."

"Is she OK now? Can I see her before I leave?"

"Of course. We gave her a shot of Acuphase, a sedative, and also one of Haldol for her psychosis. She's settled into her room now but I don't think she's asleep yet. Just don't stay long—it will only agitate her more to see you here."

"OK. It's 1:00 AM already and I have to teach school tomorrow, so I'll only stay a couple of minutes."

Kaija looked confused when I walked into her room. "Why am I in here again?" she asked.

"They didn't have a bed upstairs," I lied. "They need to get you back on antipsychotic shots again because you've been so agitated and upset. I'm sorry, darling. I don't think they'll keep you here long."

Kaija didn't argue or even appear upset. She didn't react to the doctor's term "antipsychotic" as she had always done before, nor had she mentioned platelets. She appeared defeated, and plain worn out. I hugged her and reassured her that she was in good hands here. "I know," she said. "I've been here before." I kissed her good night.

Mind Gone Astray

She responded lethargically. I walked out, alone, into the dark once again.

Week One: A Battle of Wills

I felt awful being home alone once again. I felt as though I had lost a part of myself. I did not expect this to happen again. The doctors had been so confident in their treatments at first, so hopeful, and so had I. Now I realized that my expectations had been too high, and therefore it was a severe letdown to realize that we were back at step one again. It was a good thing I was teaching school; it gave me another focus each day and enabled me to repress my feelings of guilt, self-pity, and despair that hovered just below the surface. I would have gone crazy at home alone all day.

I called the nursing station right after I got home from school. Kaija had slept through the night and for a good part of the day. The nurse suggested I not talk to her in case it would just upset her. Dr. Lewis was going to start her on Clozapine again tomorrow, I learned. It meant nothing to me. I was so confused with all the meds she had been on that I didn't remember, or even care, what this one was for.

"Kaija is still off her Clozapine," John, the nurse on duty told me the next time he phoned. "We can't force her to take it. It's not in capsule form, either, so we can't even disguise it in her food. Maybe tomorrow she'll be more compliant."

No deal. The following day she refused all her pills! She was angry, saying she only needed something for her platelets and that these pills were doing her no good. Dr. Lewis solved that by giving her another shot of Acuphase, and when that calmed her down, a shot of Respiradol. She resisted the first shot, but with the help of two nurses, they were able to administer it.

"If we can get Kaija back on Clozapine again, there's a three-week titration period," Dr. Lewis told me on the phone at the end of the week.

"What on earth does that mean?" I asked.

"It means that we need to slowly increase the dosage over three weeks and measure the concentration in her blood to see that she is reacting to the medication OK and to ensure that we don't give her more than her system will accept. We'll need to monitor her closely for negative side effects such as a decrease in white blood cells."

"You mean she'll be in there another three weeks?" I asked, incredulous.

"Yes. That's assuming we can get her to take it. We could keep giving her Haldol injections, but I'm afraid that will increase her tremors, and they're bad enough right now. Besides, it did not have the desired effect when we tried it earlier."

"Do you think the Haldol shots are responsible for her tremors?"

"It's difficult to pinpoint the cause, especially since we've tried so many different medications …"

"Well, I think it was the Seroquel. The tremors began just a few weeks after she was admitted. You had immediately stopped the Respiradol and started the Seroquel. That's when I first noticed the tremors. And they've sure become a lot worse now than they were then."

"How does Kaija explain them?"

"She just explains, matter-of-factly, that it runs in the

family, and it does on her mom's side, but usually only after they're eighty years old. One uncle, though, has had tremors most of his life. It amazes me that she accepts them so placidly."

"Well, with her being so wrapped up in her 'ad lib' world, I'm not surprised."

"I looked up tardive dyskinesia on the Internet. There it said that Propranalol is often effective in reducing tremors, but that it cannot stop them. Apparently they're irreversible. She'll have them forever, I guess …"

"Yes, she will. It's unfortunate, but it's a minor issue compared to her psychosis. We don't want to administer Propranalol while she's on antipsychotics that we're monitoring."

"Of course. I agree wholeheartedly. I wasn't suggesting you start it now. If Kaija can live with it, it's no big deal for me, either."

"That's good. Our aim now is to get the psychosis under control, and that's a challenge, as Kaija not only refused to take the Clozapine, but still refused whatever other pills we've tried to give her as well. She wouldn't even submit to a shot of Acuphase; I had to call in the guards to hold her while we gave her the injection in her hip. But I think we're slowly winning the battle," Dr. Lewis told me. "At least she's not as angry and upset as when you brought her in."

Week Two: For Better or for Worse

When I went up on Saturday, Kaija looked at me with surprise: *"I thought you were dead,"* she said.

"No, love, I'm right here. Why did you think that?"

"Those people on 'ad lib' told me."

"I wish you'd stop listening to them! Remember I told you that they all tell nothing but lies."

"Why did they take most of my clothes away?"

"I don't know, hon. Maybe they took them to wash them." What a good liar I'm getting to be, I thought. The nurse had told me when I came to the hospital that Kaija had constantly been packing them in a plastic bag, ready to go home. That's why they had taken them away, to reduce her focus on going home.

When I went to see Kaija the next day, I saw the saddest sight I have ever seen. There she sat on the side of the bed in her dingy room. She was in her winter coat, gloves on and a scarf over her head, making her look like a ninety-year-old granny. She had a haunted look in her eyes. I couldn't speak. I took her in my arms and wept and wept. She didn't ask why, but only said, in childlike innocence, *"I was waiting for you to come to take me home."*

It hurt me to the core. It was I who had brought her here to this dingy hole in the ground with its barred windows and locked doors. I could barely tolerate the situation; self-recrimination was stronger than ever before. Yet she needed help, help that I could not give.

"I'm sorry, love. I can't take you without the doctor's permission. Here, let me help you take your coat off. I'll talk to the doctor tomorrow; I don't think it will be much longer now." I couldn't control my emotions; tears kept seeping unbidden from my eyes.

As I got up to leave, Kaija said, *"I'll see you in heaven. At least there the cancer can't get you."*

I left quickly and drove all the way home. I could

have stayed in the city at Cindy's, but I just couldn't face anyone now.

Kaija's sister phoned her the next night, and then phoned me. "Kaija told me she had to get home on Sunday for your funeral," she said. "She sure has gotten worse since she went off her medications."

I could only accept and agree with that. I couldn't face going up to see her until Thursday of that week. Kaija had still refused to take her medications, but Dr. Lewis had given her an intramuscular shot of Respiradol on Tuesday. She was to get it every two weeks, I was told. This way, they hoped the drug would stay in her system longer than pills would, since she was a "high metabolizer," they reminded me.

I couldn't understand why they were trying Respiradol again, the very first drug they had tried in Riverview Hospital, but I had to believe that they were doing their best. They could only experiment until they found a drug that worked. I understood that; nevertheless, I hated the fact that it made my wife seem like a medical specimen, not the live woman she had been, and that she really was.

Kaija immediately asked me if I had come to take her home, but to my surprise, when I said "No" she accepted it placidly. We were actually able to visit. Oh, she didn't have any news to tell me and the hallucinations were still there, but she did ask how my week had gone and did tell me that she had read the *Macleans* from cover to cover. Amazing, I thought. If she was telling me the truth, that was the first reading she had done in weeks. Maybe the Respiradol was having some effect.

I took her old elementary school art portfolio up

for us to look at together the next day. We had many chuckles and I spent a delightful couple of hours with her. But when I went to leave, she became very angry and aggressive and threatened to hit me with her fist.

"It's all your fault that I can't come home! I'm going to go ask the nurse if I can go." She went, but of course the nurse told her she had to stay. I left her in tears, with an ache in my heart.

The next day, Sunday, I picked up a Caesar salad from the hospital cafeteria and ate supper with her. Kaija was in good spirits and we had an enjoyable time chatting about old times. She had not one hallucination the whole time! I hoped she would get moved upstairs and I spoke of my wishes to the nurses before I left. They promised to talk to Dr. Lewis about it.

Week Three: Plans and Preparations

I missed the entire next week of school because of the flu. Nevertheless, I forced myself to go to the city on Tuesday because it was again necessary to have an appeal hearing. This would permit the doctors in charge to detain Kaija even if she was transferred to a care home in the city or to Riverview Hospital.

The two psychiatrists at the hearing made it clear that Kaija was still gravely ill and therefore had to be detained for further treatment. One of the psychiatrists summed up her condition clearly and concisely: "Kaija has paranoid delusions, refusing her antipsychotic medicines because *'these have been taken off the market; they're harmful and dangerous.'* She believes the voices she hears telling her that these substances will kill her. She denies talking to voices, saying she just 'ad libs.' She got quite vehement and verbally abusive during the interview. She is unable to make rational decisions."

The second psychiatrist echoed these words, but added: "Multiple pharmacological options as well as twelve treatments of ECT have been tried. She is known to have hypertension and hyperthyroidism. She has recently refused all medications and has paranoid delusions regarding their use. Her psychosis is getting worse."

Of course the appeal to leave hospital was DENIED again.

I met with Dr. Lewis after the hearing.

"I thought Kaija could be moved upstairs already" were my first words to the doctor.

"She likely could be upstairs," he said, "but right now there are no beds. I don't expect that she'll be here long now, anyway. We can't keep her here indefinitely and we need to begin making some plans that would allow her to be in the hospital at Riverview, and hopefully come home from there after a week or two.

"Is she getting better, then?" I asked.

"Well, somewhat ... she thinks you're in heaven and so she hasn't been talking of going home lately. We've done another EEG and an ECG on her and the results are fine. We had her tested for Alzheimer's, too, but she scored thirty out of thirty on that test, so we can rule that out. I'm also going to confer with a top psychiatrist from New York who works with combinations of antipsychotic medications. Maybe he can give us another method of treatment that we haven't tried yet."

"So, what's the plan from here on?"

"Well, she should actually be in a rehab center or a

group home for a minimum of three months, and we want you to start looking into that. I'll talk to Dave, our social worker, and he can start looking into contacts for you. But we'll transfer her to Riverview Hospital for now."

"This whole thing seems like a merry-go-round—from hospital to home to another hospital to home ... will it ever end?"

"We're going to keep her on the Respiradol shots now that she is accepting these. She'll need to have one every two weeks. Dr. McRae can give them while she's in the hospital. Here's a copy of the Community Treatment Order that enables Riverview Hospital, and home care registered nurses—assuming she gets released to go home—to administer them. I've already filled out a transfer order and sent it to Dr. McRae and to Dr. Liu. Dr. Liu will be coming to Riverview every four or five weeks to meet with Kaija and monitor her progress."

The Community Treatment Order was careful to cover all bases, and laid things on the line:

I examined Mrs. Koivu and on the basis of this examination, I believe she
(I) is suffering from a mental disorder for which she is in need of treatment or care and supervision that can be provided in the community;

(II) has been detained in an inpatient facility for a total of sixty days or longer;

(III) as a result of the mental disorder is likely to cause harm to herself or others or to suffer substantial mental deterioration ... if she does not receive treatment and supervision in the community;

(IV) requires services in order to reside in the community;

(V) is unable to understand fully and to make informed decisions regarding her need for treatment;

(VI) is capable of complying with the requirements for treatment, and the care, under supervision, contained in this community;

and therefore the subject will be provided with the following treatment: obligatory treatment administered in the community of Respiradol Consta injections of 25–50 mg every two weeks ... and is to submit to medical treatments by the attending physician, <u>Dr. McRae</u> for a period of <u>3 months</u>, beginning on <u>November 24, 2006</u>.

Nothing new here, I thought, but I disliked the reference to Kaija as "the subject." Why did they have to use such dehumanizing terms? Wouldn't "patient" or even the name of the person be acceptable?

I went home right after the appointment, as I was feeling so lousy. I went to the local doctor in Riverview the next morning and received two shots in the butt— Benzedrine and adrenaline to overcome a bacterial reaction I had to the earlier virus. The doctor also gave me three prescriptions, one for my red and itchy rash, one antidepressant, and the third for a mood leveler, as the doctor was sure my illness had been brought on by stress.

Two mornings later, I made an appointment to talk with Cheryl Harvey, the head of Prairie West District Health Services about placing Kaija somewhere.

"I'm supposed to start looking for a care facility for Kaija," I told her, "so I thought I'd start here. You're aware that my wife has had a psychosis, aren't you, since she was first admitted to the hospital here in the summer?"

"Yes, and I just got a call from Dr. Lewis this morning

informing me of her situation and asking me to help you look into a care facility for her. Unfortunately, we don't have a variety of facilities in our health district. We have four care homes in the district, but all of them are for elderly persons who need acute care and are diagnosed at level four or five. I don't think Kaija would be in this category. Also, she would have to want to go there, and from what I gather, Kaija is pretty adamant about staying at home. We can't take patients against their will. And in any case, all of our care homes are full and we have a fairly long waiting list right now."

She seemed to be almost discouraging me, which was strange, I thought. "Kaija is retired. She's sixty-five. She has a psychosis. Wouldn't these qualify her for admission?" Not that I wanted her in an old folks home but I didn't know where else to start looking.

"The only thing we have that would help you is a respite room in the care home, which would be available for two weeks after she's released from the hospital. And that's only a short-term solution."

"Does that mean there is nothing in this area at all? Will I have to find a place in the city?"

"Maybe not. I'll put you in touch with the district mental health nurse. She works as a liaison with all the health departments in our district and I think she can give you better advice than I can and suggest some other solution. He name is Glenda McKenzie. She works out of Carsville. Her number is 306-882-5791."

Glenda came to see me the next day. She was open, friendly, and compassionate. She listened to my lament and even though she was professional in every way, I could see that she was touched by my story and concerned about my dilemma right now.

"I've talked with both Dr. Lewis and Dr. McRae, and from what they told me, I think the best option for Kaija after the hospital would be for her to be at home and have home care help you look after her. Most of the home care people are registered nurses, but some aren't. Still, Home Care can provide all kinds of services for Kaija and you right in your home. If you're at school, they can check in on her three or four times a day. They can give her her meds in the morning and at noon. They can bring hot meals or help her get a noon meal ready. If you need it, they will even come in to clean your house, or they can take Kaija to medical appointments when you're in school. They charge only $5.50 per hour or for each kind of service they perform."

"What about the Respiradol shots she's getting every two weeks?"

"There's no problem there. The RNs give them all the time."

I felt better after talking to Glenda. I liked her. She knew what she was talking about and had been able to give me concrete information to go on. And if Kaija could be at home, that would be a blessing in itself. Maybe I could even help her mental state somehow ... or better than I had been able to before.

Week Four: A Shaky Countdown

I was excited about having Kaija transferred to Riverview Hospital, and then, hopefully, home. In this frame of mind I called the Elliston Wing the next evening. My joy was soon dampened when the nurse told me that

Kaija had still not been moved out of the Dungeon and onto the second level. And she was *"getting ready to come to Charles' funeral tomorrow,"* Kaija had told the nurse. Would they even release her to Riverview? I wondered. It didn't sound like things were going well there.

I talked to Dr. Lewis the next day. "We've already spoken to the nurse in Riverview about administering the Respiradol shots. And Dr. Liu stopped in to see her today so that he will have a good idea of her condition and be able to measure any improvement."

"When will he be coming to Riverview?"

"I called Sandy McAfee this morning and set up an appointment with her and Dr. Liu for December 5 at 11:00 AM. You'll meet with them at the district health office."

"Will I have to pay for the Respiradol shots when she's out of the hospital?"

"Yes, unfortunately you will. They're covered only while she's in the hospital. And they're not cheap; they cost about four hundred dollars a shot. I'll apply to get exceptional drug status for it, but if they don't allow it, can you manage that?"

"Look, I'll do what has to be done. But I'm a bit irked if I'll have to pay for the shots when they're part of a treatment plan that is still administered by Health Care. If RNs have to give the shots, I think that they should be covered under the system."

"Well, maybe they can. I'd suggest you talk to Glenda McKenzie, the mental health nurse; she'll be able to find out the answer to that."

Glenda came by again and assured me that I would not have to pay for the Respiradol shots. She's done her

Mind Gone Astray

homework again, I thought. This lady has a lot on the ball.

"We'll set up a meeting with Kaija, Sandy, you, and me to do an assessment on what Kaija's Home Care needs will be. It's better that we do this in advance so that everyone understands the program and so things will go smoothly once she gets home. We need to remember that our goal will be to gradually create an independency, and not a dependency, and we all need to work toward that goal."

I felt as though the pieces of the puzzle were falling into place. Now if only Kaija would keep improving on these Respiradol shots …

I called her each evening after school over the next few days. I didn't hear what I wanted to—that she was happier, more content, and feeling better. The first time I called she cried most of the time. I asked her what was wrong. "Nothing," she sobbed. "I just want to come home. I thought you would be getting me today."

"Soon, hon, I'll come get you. I promise. Can you just hold out for a few more days?"

She didn't cry the next time, but sounded very despondent. *"They told me you would be getting me home at 7:00 AM tomorrow."*

On call number three she told me, *"If you don't come get me soon, the whole place would be cemented in and you'll not be able to get in to get me."*

On call number four I spoke to the nurse first. Kaija had had her scarf and coat on, ready to go home since 6:00 AM. She had even tried the door more than once and would have gone if it had not been locked. She had been angry and verbally abusive. They had started her on Celexa, an antidepressant, since she had been so despondent lately.

When I spoke to Kaija, she was in bad spirits. "I'm so frustrated in this place. I suppose I'll never get out of here! *Edward and Holly brought me four cartons of cigarettes but the nurses poked pinholes into them all and then threw them all into the garbage."*

Since Kaija was not doing well at all, I was surprised when I got a call two days later saying that I could pick her up the next day. "Come between four thirty and five o'clock because we have to set up a meeting with you and Kaija and make it very clear that this is a trial release, and to the Riverview Hospital, not to home. She needs to understand this."

So we met the next day. Everything went routinely. Kaija was quiet and subdued, but certainly eager at the same time to get out of the Dungeon. I phoned ahead to Carrie, the nurse on duty at Riverview Hospital, to tell her we would be arriving around seven thirty. It all seemed so easy now, so cut and dry, so programmed. I wasn't sure if I even felt happy, for I could not envision what this next phase would bring. It sure hadn't been peaches and cream when she had been in here before.

Chapter 11: Déjà vu

Although Kaija kept up a running chatter of hallucinations on the drive from the city—her new clothes, smoking bans in the city, dangerous road conditions, new speed limits, the names of people in the cars we met—nevertheless, she was happy and lucid when we arrived at Riverview Hospital.

"The rooms here are so bright and cheery and roomy," she told the nurses.

"We're glad to have you back," they responded warmly. "We haven't seen you for a long time."

"I'm not here to stay," replied Kaija. *"I'm just here overnight and then Charles is taking me home to our new house."*

It was déjà vu from there on. It soon became apparent to me that the old, tiring cycle was about to begin all over again: not taking meds, wanting to go home daily, eloping, having sitters with her daily, hallucinations (*"Charles is dead"*) interspersed by a few good moments.

And so it began. So that she would be less likely

to leave the hospital, the nurses gathered her coat, hat, gloves, and shoes and stored them away. When I went to visit her the first evening, she complained that *"the nurses spilled oil on all my clothes. They're all ruined so they got rid of them."*

In spite of this precaution, Kaija eloped the second day. One of the nurses saw her leaving and called for her to come back, but she didn't stop. They caught up to her just as she reached the street. *"I was just going to look at our new house,"* she said. But she came back without further argument and they gave her a shot of Haldol.

I was at a loss. What was going to happen now? I called Dr. Liu in the city.

"Get more intensive nursing staff on so that someone can watch over her constantly. If needed and possible, get family to stay with her part of the time. Draw up a schedule. We need to keep her in the hospital indefinitely now to try to give the Respiradol shots more time to work. There's no use sending her back to the city and repeating the same old cycles."

I talked to Dr. Mercer, the new doctor on Kaija's case. I asked her why Dr. McRae was not looking after Kaija as before, and was informed that Dr. McRae had too many patients already and could not take on any more at the moment. Dr. Mercer nevertheless promised to do her best.

"I tried to get more nursing staff on to help watch over Kaija" she told me the next day " but there just aren't any available. The nurses told me they're trying their best to watch her, but they can't be at the front desk all the time and Kaija could slip out easily during such times without being seen. I'm sorry. Do you have relatives and friends that could take turns staying with her?"

I hated to do it. I had always been an independent sort, perhaps because of my early farming background, or maybe just from my stubbornness to accomplish on my own whatever I wanted to do. But I realized that for my wife's safety and my own peace of mind, I'd have to comply, once again, with their request. I sat down that night and made up a list of ten relatives and close friends who could take turns being with Kaija during the days, while I would stay with her in the evenings after school. As hard as it was for me to do, I called them all that evening and set up a schedule. Later I was moved when others, after hearing of the situation, offered to spend time with her, too. My list grew to fifteen.

I scheduled my sister Janice, Kaija's sister Esther, and her sister-in-law, Lillian to take the first shifts, thinking that she would be most comfortable with them. And for the first couple of days she was. They brought in picture albums, *National Geographics, Reminisce,* and *O Canada* magazines to look through together. Occupied thus, Kaija was a model of good behavior. But it didn't last long.

When Lillian came in for the first shift, Kaija had been wild to go home. *"Let's go,"* she said every few minutes. *"Let's just go. We can walk out of here any time we want and you can take me home."* Many times she had gone to the nurses' desk to question them about when she could go, and if not, why not. She had not been taking her meds again, and it showed in her agitation and anger.

When her sister, Esther, came the next day it was a different kind of story. This time she was worried about me not getting in. *"You'd better go home because Charles is waiting in the hallway to come in, and he can't come into the room until you leave."*

Esther looked down the hall to see if indeed I was there. "I don't see any sign of him," she told Kaija. "I don't think he'll be coming until after school."

"You just can't see him because he's invisible. He's lying flat on the hall floor so he can't be seen."

When Paul, a childhood male friend came the next day, Kaija was a model of gracious behavior. She chatted with him about his family, wanting to know where all their kids were living now and what they were doing. They had coffee and a snack together in her room, and Paul afterward told me that he could detect nothing wrong with her.

But when my sister, Janice, came the next day, Kaija was extremely frustrated. *"You people don't have to be sitting watching over me every day. I know that's what you're doing. I've never run away or left once yet, so you might as well go home. I don't need to be babysat!"*

After this, the sitters remained in a lounge chair in an alcove from which they could watch both the front and side door. Sometimes Kaija would wander by, notice them, and ask what they were doing there. They had been coached to say that they were just waiting for the doctor to come, or for some blood tests to be run, or some equally white, white lie.

When, after two weeks, it eventually became apparent that Kaija was not wandering the halls as much anymore, and since she had on only her hospital garb, the hospital staff concluded that she would not elope anymore. Trial one had ended, and I felt a little less stressed.

But there were other things to worry about. Her

refusal to take many of the meds led to meetings between me and various medical personnel about how to proceed. The first meeting included Dr. Mercer, Sarah Persson, the hospital and Home Care administrator, Cheryl Harvey, the head of Prairie West District Health Services, my sister Janice (a registered nurse), a secretary to keep minutes, and me.

The minutes first summarized the current state of Kaija's condition:

> Staff at Riverview Hospital are seeing limited improvements. Kaija is making some eye contact. She is still not taking all of her meds but has been sleeping better with Lorazepam. She continues to refuse to take Loxapine, another antipsychotic begun recently. She is also on Benztropine, which is given to counteract the side effects of the antipsychotic. She has been started on 25 mg of Trazedone, which is an antidepressant and has been found to be useful with clients who wander. To date we have not seen a difference but we hope for improvement.

I felt my head beginning to swim with all the medication names, but at least the doctor explained generally what they were for.

The minutes then expressed Janice's concerns:

> If Kaija is able to return home, I'm afraid that Charles will be overloaded. Last time she was at home there was an escalation in her refusal to do most things from getting meals or cleaning house, to going out walking or visiting or whatever. She also harassed Charles hourly about moving to the nonexistent new house, to the point that he became very stressed. Kaija wanders because she has this imaginary home in her mind and she wants to meet Charles there. Charles has tried to minimize this by having no bags, boxes, or suitcases in the house.

The report went on to mention the difficulty and stress of providing daily sitters, the continuing hallucinations, and the difficulties in administering meds. A plan was then developed to deal with future needs:

1. Sarah Persson will try to find special care aides who are not scheduled for work to cover for a few days.
2. A GAU (Gerontology Assessment Unit) examination will be scheduled to consider natural aging processes as contributing factors. (Humbug, I thought, she's not eighty years old!)
3. Glenda McKenzie will be asked to determine, with help as needed, whether we are dealing with psychosis or dementia. (Kinda late to be ruling this out, I thought).
4. Dr. Mercer will apply for exceptional drug cost status to minimize costs once Kaija is out of hospital.
5. If wandering or eloping continues, we will try to access a convalescent bed in a secure facility such as in Elmwood. (I did not like that one, as Elmwood was almost a two-hour drive away.)
6. Charles asked that Dr. Lewis still be in Kaija's circle of care even though Dr. Liu will be coming to see her in Outlook, because Kaija has built up a strong trust relationship with Dr. Lewis. Dr. Mercer said she would look into this.
7. Should the decision be made to release Kaija to her home, a home care assessment will be done and services set in place as needed to support her and Charles. These may include: (a) Home Care RNs giving daily medications, (b) in-home meal prep two to three times a week to ensure proper nutrition, and (c) in-home respite for Charles to get away for a break, as needed. (Oh, I needed one all right, but would my guilt ever let me take one?)

I felt somewhat relieved after the meeting. I didn't like the parts that focused on me, though, for it seemed to me that their concern was misdirected. So what if I was a little burned out? I'd manage. It had been a long time since Kaija had last been home, and I was excited about her finally, maybe, being released. I was hopeful, anyway. No one could take my hope away from me. Lately, it had often seemed that even that was being torn from me, yet every time Kaija showed even a little improvement, my heart lifted. Yes, perhaps somewhat guardedly, after having had my hope shattered so many times. But the Scottish proverb "Were it not for hope, the heart would break" certainly was true. Hope had carried me this far and had won over despair. I'd not give up.

As if in answer to my silent prayers, Kaija had three good days in a row. When I visited the first evening after the meeting, she actually conversed with me about the day's happenings at the hospital and asked me about my day at school. I was amazed that she did not once mention going home. It was the best evening I had spent with her by far.

The next two evenings she was not quite so talkative, but even though her conversation was minimal, it was lucid. I learned from the night nurse that they had had sitters there for the days but that they did not feel they needed them to be there anymore. Kaija had been pleasant, had come to the desk to talk with them a number of times, and had walked in the halls for exercise quite often. Was she actually improving, or was this just a blip on the screen again? I hated myself for being doubtful.

The next night shattered any hopes that the improvements were significant or lasting. Kaija was in a state of torment and battered me with a continual barrage of *"Let's go home ... we can go now ... you don't want me at home ... Dr. Mercer is invisible in the hall—she says we can go ... You said you'd take me home as soon as you get back from heaven ..."*

I felt the despair rising to the surface again. This was magnified when the nurse gave me a copy of the discharge paper that had finally come to the hospital from Dr. Lewis. I took it home and began reading it. They detailed everything: a "history of her illness," past psychiatric history of depression, past medical history (hyperparathyroidism, hypertension, osteoarthritis, mitral stenosis, fibromyalgia), past surgical history (appendectomy, carpal tunnel, hysterectomy, radical mastectomy for breast cancer), family history (positive for depression and one cousin with schizophrenia) as well as "social history"(no children) ... retired ... lately decreased motivation and lack of energy ... smokes twelve cigarettes a day and justifies this because she has *"mitral stenosis"* ... uses no alcohol or street drugs ...

My poor, poor darling, I thought. I knew she had some tough times in her life, but to have them all spelled out like this one after another shocked me. It seemed to me that our life together had been rich and fulfilling, and that we had weathered these tougher moments well. Our love for one another had carried us through, and had lightened the strains of the trying times. I had never thought of my wife as sickly, for her major health problems had come and gone, come and vanished with the operations. Well, that was true except for her arthritis and fibromyalgia; these had for sure been ongoing and

Mind Gone Astray

taxing. I wondered if they, over many long years, had contributed to some degree to her present mental state.

The "MENTAL STATUS EXAMINATION" was nothing but depressing, even though I had long now known its highlights: "Sixty-five-year-old female looking older than her age ... taken directly from her home by ambulance. Affect appeared irritable and flat. She denied any visual hallucinations, but she admits to having auditory hallucinations. She also had somatic hallucinations, believing that the pain in her leg is caused by people poking her. She had paranoid delusions regarding her prescribed medications saying 'all the mood stabilizers have been taken off the market.' Judgment was limited by delusions, and insight was poor."

What damning evidence of a sick, sick girl! I had lived through all this. Again it seemed to me even more terrible to have it compacted this way into one written paragraph! Was it that experience could be forgotten, wiped out, whereas the written word was preserved and brooked little or no argument? I thought of the Nazi book burnings—the attempt to try to destroy the truth, the past, in this way! I knew that my memory was not great, did not even hold a candle to Kaija's. I knew that the bad was often repressed and forgotten and that in a life unscarred by trauma, the good memories usually survived. I suddenly felt angry—why did they have to document every little thing and throw it in my face this way?

The torture continued. "COURSE IN HOSPITAL: Kaija was noncompliant with medications during her hospitalization ... Despite treatment she continued to have low moods and to be irritable. She also continued to have paranoid delusions, refusing medication and being distrustful of medical personnel. At times she would start crying, saying that her husband had died of appendicitis, or heart failure, or cancer, and that he would have to be buried in the next few days. When confronted about her delusions, she would always be either nonchalant or aggressive."

Surely this was not my wife described here! But I could not escape the truth of the written word, and I wept and wept until there were no tears left.

The "DISCHARGE PLAN" was matter-of-fact and neutral in tone: "Kaija was transferred to Riverview Hospital under Dr. Mercer's care ... the treatment will be supervised by Glenda McKenzie, and Dr. Jin Min Liu is going to see Kaija at the clinics in Riverview. There is a possibility that Kaija will be transferred back to City Hospital if elopement risk becomes more visible."

The killing blow came suddenly at the end of the report: "THERE IS ALSO AN APPLICATION FOR THE MENTAL INSTITUTION IN SOUTH BORDEN AS A FUTURE OPTION FOR KAIJA."

I knew of this institution. It was the last one left in the province. Most of them had been closed down years ago when they were deemed "ineffective in treating most mentally ill clients" and the patients were moved into smaller group homes. This one was for the most severe cases—those who were hard to control and for whom typical treatment just did not work, or for those who had to be locked up because of criminal records.

Long ago, Dr. Lewis had told me that this was the final alternative if all else failed. I had repressed it, forgotten all about it. It just had not seemed possible that Kaija would ever be diagnosed as such a severe case. Yet here was the possibility, in writing, staring me in the face. I felt numb. It would never happen! I would sacrifice all I had, all my energy, all my happiness to prevent it. No matter how difficult it might become to keep her at home, I would do it. Never, never, never would I let it happen!

Tentatively, the Health Care workers and I tested the waters over the next few days. A pass to go to church on Sunday. Another to go to the city for an eye appointment and to shop on Tuesday. An evening and night at home on Thursday, but back in for injection and observation Friday. Kaija wept at having to go back, but did not get angry or abusive.

Kaija was in good spirits during each brief pass. She returned and initiated comments—lucid ones, most of the time. She was interested in talking to friends at church, actually excited about shopping for new clothes, and very, very happy all during the evening at home. In the hospital, the nurses told me, she was pleasant, made no attempts to leave, and took her Respiradol shots willingly. Dr. Liu had been in to see her and she had agreed that she should stay on the program of medications so that she could go home to stay.

School ended for me on Friday, December 23. On Saturday, Kaija came home! The past six month's trials vanished in my happiness.

Chapter 12: Episodic Nightmare

"Why are we going here?" asked Kaija as I pulled into the driveway. *"I thought we were going to the new house. Dr. Naipaul and the family are all waiting there."*

Oh, no, I groaned inwardly. Don't tell me it's going to be the same as last time. And Kaija had been so good the past few days: few hallucinations, generally happy, somewhat quieter than her usual self, yes, but still lucid, responsive, with light in her eyes.

"This is where we live, hon. We don't have a new house. And Dr. Naipaul was my heart doctor, remember. He lives in the city. I haven't seen him since my last checkup a year ago."

She didn't argue, but I could see she had her own thoughts about that.

"When are you going to go for your insulin shot?" she asked as soon as we were inside.

"I don't have diabetes, hon. Where did you get that idea?"

"You do so, and you know it, too!"

It was my turn to not argue. I was tired, so I decided to have a nap on the couch. Kaija went upstairs to lie on the bed and rest. But as I lay on the sofa, five times in half an hour Kaija came down, saying, *"Let's go get your insulin shot."* Once, as I was about to doze off, I became aware of her carefully feeling my jeans' pockets. *"Do you have a syringe so you can give yourself a shot of insulin?"* she asked.

I simply ignored her and pretended I was asleep. Five minutes later she was back. *"You'd better get up because Glen Thurston is upstairs doing his banking on our computer."* I rose and went with her upstairs.

"Look, there's no one here," I said as we entered the study.

"He's here but he's invisible."

"Well, let him be. He won't do any harm. Let's just listen to some music for a while." Whenever I could, I would try to divert Kaija's thoughts to something else. It often worked and she'd forget about that particular hallucination altogether.

That evening began what was to become a ritual every night as Kaija got ready for bed. As before, she'd lock the bathroom door, shut off the lights, and begin to wash up and get ready for bed. The difference from last time was that for up to ten minutes I would hear her talking loudly and vehemently to her various voices. I couldn't do anything about her bathroom conversations, however. She usually emerged angry, frustrated, and hurt to the point of tears.

After this, or a similar diatribe each evening, Kaija became quiet and calm. She put on her pajamas, crawled into bed, and lay totally still, except for an extreme tremor in her left hand. When she lay her arm across my chest, her hand would "thump, thump, thump" against me, but I didn't let it bother me. It felt good just to have her there beside me. Gradually, the tremor lessened and she relaxed. Sometimes she would ask me to forgive her for losing her temper, and I would bless her. She was comforted by this, as was I. At least her faith had not been shaken and lost in the turmoil of her mind, I thought. It comforted me. It just goes to show that mind and spirit are not one bit the same thing, I thought. In my heart I knew that, but I had greatly feared that such mental trauma might blur the distinction for her.

Christmas Eve went well. We picked up her father, Mika, from the retirees' home and went to Lars and Lillian's. Kaija had no hallucinations but she was subdued, had a somewhat haunted look in her eyes, and had little to add to the conversation. But she seemed to enjoy watching her little nephews and nieces opening their gifts.

Christmas day she was much the same while we were at Esther and Walter's. But the day didn't start out that way: *"Dad's tied down in his bed. Lars and Lillian just told me on 'ad lib.'"*

"That's not true! Why do you listen to those voices?"

"It is so. You heard them, too. Why don't you listen sometime!"

Kaija would not believe me, so I suggested she phone Esther and ask her. She did. After Esther reassured her that Mika was not tied down, she replied not a word but simply hung up. *"Lars and Lillian lied to me,"* she said angrily. *"I'm never going there again!"*

The afternoon went well, but Kaija was quiet and

subdued, and I could see that she was on edge the whole time. Only when we feasted on the turkey dinner did she appear to let go and actually enjoy herself. After dinner, as she sat on the sofa, I could tell that she was not following the conversations at all, and two or three times I saw her lips moving. She was conversing, all right, but not with anyone in the room.

On Monday morning I awoke to her weeping. *"These voices are constantly tormenting me—they just won't quit. 'Ad lib' is the in thing now, so everybody's on it and I can't ever shut them off."*

Sad, sad, sad! I felt so helpless, so tormented myself by her tormented state. If the voices just weren't so rampant and critical! It puzzled me that she spoke about the voices, indicating that she knew, or at least sensed, that she had an illness, a problem other than her platelets, as she usually said; however, at the same time she seemed totally unaware of her seamless transitions from reality to hallucination. Or was it that she just could not bring herself to admit that she had a mental illness? "No insight" is what the doctors called it. Was this classic repression? It was the only answer that made any sense to me.

When the Home Care nurse came to give Kaija her injection the next morning, she commented, "Look, she even has a smile for me this morning." And indeed she did. She had life in her eyes, too, and after the nurse left she sorted out two loads of clothes all on her own and put them to wash. A major accomplishment, I thought. She had done nothing at all since coming home, had not even helped with meals or putting the dishes into the dishwasher.

But the major accomplishment was soon to be wiped

out by what I deemed a major episode. It was to be the first of many. I was so taken aback, so upset, that I recorded each episode in a journal. If this was a turning point for the worse, a regression, I needed to date them and remember them when I next talked to the psychiatrist.

Episode One: Tuesday, December 26, 2006
I went upstairs after lunch one day, and there I found Kaija curled up in fetal position on the floor in her clothes closet. The folding doors were almost shut, leaving only a narrow opening out of which she was peering. I was shocked. I had never seen her like this before. She was obviously feeling paranoid; it wasn't the first time, but before she had answered her critics and her tormenters in anger, full voice, aggressive. Never had she withdrawn or hidden from them like this. I felt sick with dread.

"My poor honey, what are you doing lying in the closet like that?" I asked.

"I'm hiding here so Lars will quit poking me in the chest and leg. I can't get him to leave me alone. But he can't find me in here.

"Are you in pain somewhere, hon?" I wondered if her fibromyalgia was bothering her again and this was how she explained the pains.

"Only when he pokes me." She then launched into a long and loud outburst in Finnish, angrily responding to a number of people, as far as I could tell. She rattled on in Finnish so fast that I could hardly follow what she was saying. Then she went on and on about all kinds of things. I can't even remember what they were, but the one that sticks in my mind is, *"God says I told you to go to hell. Have I ever said that?"*

I helped her out of the closet and held her close. She was trembling and sobbing now, like a child afraid of the dark. She clung to me and I just held her tight for a long time. When she finally stopped weeping, I told her to lie on the bed. I tucked her under a heavy quilt, thinking that would give her a sense of security. I then got her two Ativan, and lay down on the bed with my arm around her. I couldn't help it—I wept as I held her. She asked me why I was crying, and I told her that I was crying for her, not for me. A bit later she asked me to forgive her for her anger and for distressing me. I could only weep more, but I blessed her, as she did me. I wonder—who was the comforter here?

* * *

Since my year of teaching had been a contract job, replacing a regular teacher who was on maternity leave, I was now out of work. There just were no teaching jobs to be had this January. It didn't bother me, though. I figured that if I could get employment insurance for a few months, I'd be able to stay home with Kaija, to watch over her. Even more important, I wanted to try to bring her out of her inner self, to help diminish the horrible hallucinations and the constant torment of the voices in her head, and gently lead her back into real life again. I wasn't sure how I was going to accomplish this, but I had rolled around in my mind various ways of stimulating her and was determined to do whatever I could to help her.

The next morning as I sat at the computer filling out an application for EI, I could hear Kaija talking loudly in the bedroom. It was hard for me to concentrate. I tried to block it out, but the thought kept eating at me, "That's my wife in there!" It was ironic. Kaija was the one who was unable to distinguish unreality from reality, yet here I was, unable myself to come to grips with the reality that this lady was indeed my wife.

Even Kaija's body structure had withered to that of an eighty-year-old because she had lost so much weight. When she walked, she shuffled along like one twenty years older than she actually was. Both mind and body had suffered such debilitating effect over the past two years that even both our families were horrified. They just could not understand what had happened to their sister/sister-in-law over the past two years. First the virus with its continual bouts of diarrhea for over six months, then eight months of depression, and finally this!

It seemed to me that the virus she had contacted while we were in China teaching ESL was the culprit that had started it all. Some of the literature suggested that in some cases a virus could possibly be one of the many causes of some psychoses, but Kaija's doctors seemed to place little weight on this when I mentioned it to them. But they, too, were still shaking their heads, and although they had tried to categorize the illness so that they would know exactly what they were treating, they were really still just experimenting with medications to treat symptoms that were common to many different mental illnesses.

I managed to bring my mind back on track—until the loud talking turned into weeping. That I could not ignore, so I went in to see what was wrong.

Episode Two: Wednesday, December 27, 2006

As I was trying to concentrate on filling out my EI application via the Internet, I heard Kaija weeping in our bedroom. Again she was curled up in a ball, this time on the bed, rocking gently back and forth. When I tried to comfort her, she suddenly sat up and shouted at me, *"Dr. Naipaul is waiting for us at the new house and you just sit there on the computer! What are you doing, anyway?"*

"I'm filling out my application for EI," I said.

"I don't know why you're bothering with that. We have two million dollars in the bank."

"No, hon, we don't. And we don't have a new house, either."

That's when she hit me. It didn't have much force behind it, and she just slugged me on the shoulder. Nevertheless, it was the first time she had ever struck me in all our married life. I was taken aback, yet oddly, I was amused at the same time for her attempts were so feeble, so futile. David and Goliath, I thought. Perhaps I even smiled a bit at this thought and at the pathos in her attacking me in her weak state. She saw this and she fumed in anger, *"You never believe me! I could almost hate you! We do so have a new house,"* and she pounded me on the shoulder four more times. I don't think she wanted to hurt me because then she would have lashed out at my face. She was just so frustrated with me for always negating her "truths" that she just had to get through to me somehow.

"Look, hon, if we had a new house, do you think I'd be sitting here and not moving? I'd like a new house, too, instead of having to rent this duplex. But this is where we live now; it's comfortable and we should be happy that it's such a nice, cozy place."

That's when she grabbed the cordless telephone and bopped me over the head. Again, not hard, but with a clear intent to drive some sense into my mind! I couldn't help it—I laughed outright. It was a scene right out of the comic strip, "Pickles."

"Come on, hon, you don't hate me that much," I said. She looked at me as though she herself was amazed at what she had done. She looked a little afraid, too, likely wondering how I would react. I took the phone away from her, gathered her in my arms, and held her close. I expected her to resist, but she didn't. Instead she clung to me, as if afraid I would leave. A hug is so therapeutic. She stopped crying immediately and I was able to divert her thoughts by suggesting we have some lunch.

I hope this is not going to continue! Physical aggression is taboo in today's world, and if the Home Care nurses ever see it, or worse, become the object of it, there will be an immediate uproar and Kaija will be hospitalized again toute de suite. I don't want that!

* * *

The next few days were uneventful, other than the fact that Kaija had lots and lots of hallucinations. And delusions. One night, as we lay in bed, she talked for a long time in a quiet voice to *Taivaan Valtion Isa* (the Heavenly Father), she told me when I asked. This grandiosity is really taking hold, I thought. Even though it was a common symptom, it remained so very strange to my rational mind. As usual, there were also conversations about getting boxes to pack for the move to the new house, Dr. Mercer *"nattering"* at her every time she had a smoke, and people poking at her sore leg. But there were a couple of new ones, too.

"I don't have a sore throat," she shouted one day.

"Who said you did?" I asked.

"Dr. Mercer and Lars both said so. Just because when I swallow it makes a little noise doesn't mean it's sore. They always think they know everything."

Another time it was, *"I can't even fly anymore because of the gold in my back."*

There were no more instances of what most people would term 'physical abuse,' but what to me were only my honey communicating to me in sign language what she couldn't get me to understand verbally.

Episode Three: Thursday, December 28, 2006
Another major episode today, in the evening. Kaija became obsessed with the notion that Brady (wherever she picked up that name, I'll never know) was concerned about my supposed diabetes. At least ten times within a half hour after we had gone to bed she said to me, *"Brady's coming over to give you your insulin shot."*

Mind Gone Astray

"I don't have diabetes, hon," I said to her gently. However my gentleness did not last beyond the fifth denial. I became more and more stressed out and impatient, more and more vehement, finally asking in exasperation, "Wherever did you get that strange idea? I've never had diabetes in my life, so I wish you'd quit talking about it!" I'm sure I sounded angry, and I immediately regretted losing my cool.

Kaija didn't reply. But if the repetition got to me, which it did, it was nothing compared to what was to come. After my outburst I went downstairs, but I hadn't even reached the bottom step when I heard the most pitiful wailing, keening, that I have ever heard. *"Ooijiiiaaa ... aaaahoijaa ... aaaaah ... aaiijiii ... niiinii ... aaa ... aaiijii!"* It seemed to come from deep within her and to express a misery that knew no bounds. I thought of the soul-wrenching keening of the aboriginal women, long ago, when their warrior husbands had been killed in battle, or of the Rwandan (and others) wives whose husbands and children were killed before their eyes by rebel guerilla warriors. I had never heard the sound, but in my imagination it lived powerfully and epitomized, for me, the very depths of despair. Now, for the first time, I heard the sound. At first I wasn't even sure what it was, and it is impossible to accurately describe it; perhaps it could be called a high-pitched, long, drawn moan of pain—pain in the heart. It shocked me into immobility and shook me to my core. "She's really gone crazy now" were the words that flashed through my mind.

I stood rooted to the spot, heart thumping, listening, not knowing if I dared go up to try to comfort her or if it was better to leave her alone with her grief for a while. For five long minutes I stood there, guilt-ridden, anguished, hating myself for losing my temper. I couldn't escape the knowledge that it had been my boorish behavior that had brought this on. How I must have hurt her! Never, in all our life, had I heard such a terrible sound. *"Aaaaah ... aaiijiii ... niiinii ... aaa ... aaiijii."* It etched itself into my mind.

It subsided, eventually. I crept quietly up the stairs. Kaija was sitting on the side of the bed, hunched over, head almost to her knees, and rocking slowly back and forth. I went over and took her in my arms. She submitted to being held like a little child. I just held her. What could I say? An apology seemed so shallow. I had hurt her to the core, yet here she was in my arms, seeking comfort when I was too shattered to even give her any. I lay her down on her pillow and tucked her in.

For a long time we both lay there, silence between us. Then she got up and went downstairs, for a drink of water I supposed. "What did you go down for?" I asked her.

"I went to let Brady in, but he was invisible so he couldn't get in."

Three times within ten minutes she did this. I told her to not worry, that Brady had gone home now and that we could see about it in the morning. I finally found the strength to ask her to forgive me. She seemed confused for a moment, as if trying to grasp what I had asked her to do and why. Then she gently put her arm around my neck and said, "Don't cry. I forgive you, in Jesus name and blood, for whatever you have done. Be comforted. God sees you and he forgives you, too."

* * *

The next day Kaija seemed to have undergone a transformation, as though whatever had been bothering her had been purged. Not once did she mention the diabetes, or Dr. Naipaul, or the new house. She didn't want to take her Respiradol shot from the Home Care nurse at first, but when she was encouraged to "stay on the course and take your meds because that's the only thing that will make you better," she submitted.

The rest of the day she was very tired. She talked with some of her voices, but very quietly and only intermittently. She showered and got ready for bed without a single angry outburst, not even locking the door or turning the light off. I washed her hair and her back for her. She was grateful for this, as always.

For the next few days life seemed almost normal. There were hallucinations, as always, but only intermittently. She began to read the *Daily Post*—not very much of it, but it was the first sign of interest she had shown of news in the outside world. One day we went for a short walk—only two blocks, but it was another breakthrough. We even worked on a jigsaw puzzle that I had set up before she came home, in the hope that it would divert her from her inner mind and give us something to do together.

But soon I could sense the anxiety building up in her again. One afternoon as she was lying on the sofa she suddenly said, *"Honest to Pete! I can't even lie down the right way to please anyone anymore!"*

A few minutes later it was, *"I've never felt so discouraged. These 'ad lib' voices just keep cursing me all day long."*

Was this a beginning of what the psychiatrists called "insight," this outright admission that there were voices in her head? It wasn't the first time I, or the doctors either for that matter, had heard her mention her voices, but this time she appeared to be so with it and so naturally angry at their intrusion on her life, on reality. For some reason, the opening line of an old song began to spin round and round in my head: "I can see clearly now, the rain is gone." I wished I could see clearly inside her head. If I could, I'd sure block these crazy, insistent voices out for her. But as always, I felt helpless and could only commiserate with her in a wholly ineffectual way.

Another day, again while lying on the sofa, she exclaimed to me, *"He's not even a human being! I have no use for him at all! I'm never going to visit there again."*

"Who are you talking about?"

"You heard him—that stupid cousin of mine, Delbert."

"Sorry, hon, I told you I can't hear or talk on 'ad lib.' If you think I'm on there, you're wrong. It's just someone impersonating me. And remember I told you that everything on 'ad lib' is lies?"

"Well, I thought you were on there and heard him."

"Well, I didn't. What did he say?"

"He's such an ass. He's mad at me for reading a novel. He says I should read two of the Voice of Zion papers first."

Kaija got up, went upstairs and got two of the magazines, settled back on the sofa, and began to read. She didn't get far, however, when she quipped, *"How come he can swear? He's a pastor. He's just a good-for-nothing guy."*

It was the next day that the fourth major kerfuffle occurred, over such a simple thing as the thermostat setting.

Episode Four: Monday, December 31, 2006

Kaija woke me at 11:30 PM. *"You'd better go downstairs and turn our thermostat lower because if ours is too high, the landlady's side gets very hot. It's thirty degrees in her place now."*

"How do you know that?" I asked her.

"Because you can feel the heat on her side right through this wall."

I made no move to go, so Kaija got up to go and *"turn our thermostat down to sixteen degrees."*

"Don't you go down there!" I said sharply. She got back into bed and I told her to stop listening to those voices. She lay there, silent for a long time. Then, just as I was dozing off, she asked, *"Where is that furnace switch? I'm going down to turn it off."*

I lost it and yelled at her: "Quit worrying about the heat. I'll go down and fix it so you'll have some peace of mind.

Mind Gone Astray

And me too!" So I went down, but did not do anything; the thermostat was set at eighteen degrees and that was perfect for sleeping. When I went back up, she was putting on her housecoat "to go down for a smoke."

"I might as well go with you," I said. "I sure can't sleep now." I was sure she wanted to go just to see if she could find a furnace switch to shut it off. That would be all we needed—a furnace shut off and a temperature of ten degrees in the morning!

She did look carefully at all sides of the furnace while I pretended not to notice. When she could not find a switch, she sat beside me to have a smoke, not saying a word. I tried to convince her once again that the voices were false, but it was like talking to a dead air space. I don't know if she even heard me; she just sat there, not looking at me, not answering.

What might she try next? I wondered. Where was her mind now? What were the voices telling her to do? I soon found out. After I had crawled back into bed, she soon followed.

"I propped the outside door open so Karl can get in to fix the furnace, even if we're asleep."

"For heaven's sake, we'll freeze in here," I exclaimed, and went down to shut the door. This acting upon her impulses—or more accurately, in response to the "ad lib" voices—scared me. This was how things had first started out: first the eloping from Riverview Hospital, later the packing of bags and suitcases to take to the new house, making coffee for visitors that would never come ... There were endless possibilities. Waking up in a freezing cold house would have been a minor issue compared to the countless scenarios I conjured up in my mind—scenarios in which she was in danger, in agony over an injury, or even dead.

I no sooner got back into bed than Kaija said, *"Go down and unlock the door so Karl Robinson can get in. He came to fix the furnace now."*

"Listen, hon, it's already one o'clock. He sure wouldn't be coming in the middle of the night. Besides, there's nothing wrong with the furnace."

"I suppose he's just supposed to kick the door down when he gets here then ... Oh, he just said he's not coming ... No, there he is, waiting at the door now ..."

I went downstairs, ostensibly to let Karl in. I got two of my Clonazepam antianxiety pills, and took them up to her. The diatribe, however, continued, so I came downstairs to sleep on the La-Z-Boy. I pulled it across the entry to the kitchen so that if she came down to try to shut the furnace off, she'd not be able to get by me.

Kaija didn't come downstairs, but after a while she hollered at me from the top of the stairs: "Do you want your long johns and slippers?" She must have thought I'd be cold downstairs. I took this for a sign that she was back in the real world again, even if only momentarily, and drifted off. It was a horrible and short sleep.

* * *

So ended the year—horribly! Unlike my sleep, it had been a long and seemingly endless one. I felt as though two years had been crammed into the past seven months. It had been the end of May when the lockdown of Kaija's mind all started. Since then, Kaija had been in Riverview Hospital a total of 41 days, and in the Elliston psychiatric ward for 133 days. It felt like it had been forever.

Chapter 13: A Glimmer of Light

January 1—a new year ... a new hope? Well, the last few days extinguished any flicker of hope I had that now that Kaija was home to stay, things would be better. The episodes that had finished off the year had destroyed my optimism once again.

Still, my hope would not die. Any little sign of life would reawaken it, and fortunately so, for it kept me from sinking into despair.

Strangely, the new year brought signs of an awakening in Kaija—not any amazing changes or improvements, but little signs that led me to think that perhaps she was on the road to recovery. Was it going to be Frost's "road less traveled by"? Was there going to be any difference? Yes, she first refused to take her Citalopram from the Health Care nurse the first morning, telling me, *"If I die, you will be to blame."* But she eventually did take it, and from then on, she had by far her best day yet since coming home. She rested peacefully in the morning, and smiled three or four times as I was conversing with her. And she actually laughed once! That was a first!

In the afternoon we worked on the jigsaw puzzle of a Chinese pagoda in the bright afternoon sunshine flowing through the large living room window. It was fun. Kaija herself suggested she make supper—another first. The pork chops, browned and fried in Golden Mushroom soup, were yummy. After supper we went for a fairly long walk, yet another first, and in the evening I got her to play three games of Yahtzee. She did end the day with a comment about going *"to the new house with Dr. Naipaul tomorrow,"* but when I did not respond, she fell peacefully asleep.

The following day a number of repetitive hallucinations reoccurred, but for the first day since coming home she did not mention the "new house." Even if hallucinations would fade one at a time, I thought, I could live with that. Slow progress, maybe, but progress nevertheless.

Early in January, I took Kaija to the city for a geriatric assessment. I wasn't even sure what that was all about, but the dictionary informed me that geriatrics was "the branch of medicine that deals with the diseases and hygiene of old age." If they were concerned about this, why hadn't they done such an assessment a long time ago? Perhaps because she was only in her early sixties (not eighties as she appeared) they had not considered it necessary. But since she now looked so much older because of her physical deterioration, and because the psychiatrists were still seeking a cause for her psychosis, they must have decided to test her out, just to rule out dementia.

Similar to the psychiatric reports, this one was long and detailed. It covered her personal history, her family history, and a review of her "systems," including energy level, vision, hearing, dentures, appetite, past injuries, and of course the long list of her past medical history including that of the present. A few sentences caught my attention: "She is not suicidal; family history is positive for depression on her mother's side, and dementia in old age ... She is very independent in toilet, feeding, dressing, grooming ... She very much depends on her husband for shopping, food preparation, housekeeping, and financial matters.

One sentence stuck out: "There is no physical violence from her side." Did that imply that there was from my side, or was it just a standard phrase? Good thing they didn't know about the episode with the telephone! I thought.

The report detailed the condition of her head and neck, respiration, chest, abdomen, nervous system, pupils, hearing, muscle tone, limb sensation, reflex, coordination, gait, etc. All these were normal for her age, the report noted. I was relieved that, although she appeared to have aged significantly since the onset of the viral infection, she was nevertheless in relatively good physical health.

Not so positive were the statements that followed: "CT scan shows some microvascular changes during her stay at City Hospital ... High parathyroid level and low vitamin D level, but checked by endocrinologist at that time." I had not been informed of the microvascular changes or the high parathyroid level. I wondered why not, but I supposed that they were not significant enough to warrant any treatment. Nevertheless, part of the recommendations at the end of the report stated:

"It would be worthwhile to be checked by one of the internists or neurologists regarding her high parathyroid level and tremor ... I suggest a small dose of Propranolol be tried for her essential tremor." What the word "essential" meant I did not know. The literature simply described it as "tardive dyskinesia," and explained that it could sometimes be reduced, but never eliminated. Sad, I thought.

That was another thing I had wondered about many times—the tremor or actual shaking in her left hand. However, when I asked Dr. Lewis about it, I was bluntly told, again, "We can look into that later." Dr. Lewis had earlier assured me that the development of a tremor was never the side effect of ECT, and I was still convinced that it had been caused by the Seroquel.

I decided that, based on Kaija's present condition—that is, essentially no improvement—I would still not push the Propranolol issue. Since it did not cause any embarrassment for Kaija, it didn't bother me either, though for her sake, I wished it wasn't there. It made it impossible for her to crochet, the hobby that she had learned from her grandma. Not only that, she could barely sign her name, and though she tried reading, she could not hold the paper or magazine still.

Then followed all kinds of "medicalese" that I could not understand at all, details such as, "Her mini-mental is 28/30, MOCA is 28/30, and SMS is 95/100." There was a whole long paragraph similar in technical language, but I picked out the word "normal" in two or three places so I assumed all this was just routine and everything was OK.

To my delight, Kaija scored very high on all the

cognitive tests. The report noted that "she is a lady with a high level of function in computers and she loves to be involved in some type of activity." Not only that, she scored in the top 1 percent in memory! That was my honey! That was the girl with whom I had spent over forty wonderful years! I was glad they did the assessment. It showed me that not all was lost, and it gave me confidence and courage to go on battling this thing that had intruded on our lives. My hopes revived, again.

I decided not to look for another teaching job in the spring semester. I had anticipated Kaija's return home after Christmas already in November, and the plans of moving her back to Riverview Hospital for two weeks was a transition step toward her coming home to stay. Dr. Lewis had made it clear that she could be at home only under my supervision, and with the help of Home Care as needed, especially in administering the meds. I had concurred. I was more than willing to stay at home so that I could, perhaps, slowly bring her out of the unreal world in her head and back into reality. Oh, I knew that I could not cure her any more than the psychiatrists and other Health Care personnel could. Still, if I could just help her to fight off her paranoia from those voices and help her find some delight in each day, that was all I expected for the time being. "The recovery process in these kinds of cases is sometimes very long," I had been told numerous times already. "Usually it's months, and sometimes even years. And the degree of recovery can never be predicted; it differs with each patient."

Even though I knew this, I was optimistic. There had been those few days when Kaija was almost normal for long periods of time. And now this GAU report did much to raise my hopes. Perhaps it was a naive reaction. Perhaps I just hoped so hard that I blocked out any other possibility other than that she would get well—at least well enough so that we could be together as husband and wife again and enjoy life, even with the many adjustments I knew there would be.

Another positive sign to me was that she seemed to be coming to some awareness of her true illness—that the problem was a mental one, not just a physical one about *"sticking platelets."* There were no overt admissions of such, but she complained a number of times over the next few days about actual voices in her head, as opposed to talking on "ad lib" as she usually explained it up till now.

One evening when she was again tormented by these voices, she commented, "Oh, hon, it seems that our life has turned upside down, and it's all because of these voices bothering me."

Another time, as she was going through her bathroom ritual and vehemently telling the critical voices to *"shut up,"* she came out and said to me, "I go to the bathroom and even though I lock the door, I can't get away from these voices."

When I came home from church one Sunday, Kaija was looking confused and forlorn. "What's the matter, love? Why do you look so unhappy?" I asked.

"You didn't bring me my medicine, did you? I've been waiting for hours. If I don't get it, the RCMP will come and take me into the hospital for three months!"

Fear of incarceration in a hospital or worse, a mental institution of some kind, was definitely the catalyst for many of these kinds of statements. She knew of the one, the only remaining large institution in the province, that had only the worst cases in it.

One time when she was weeping, I asked, "Why are you crying so hard?"

"Because all these voices in my head woke me up. *First Calvin and then Lars told me to get busy and do something or I'd end up in an asylum. I've heard that so many times from so many people.*"

"It's OK, hon. Don't even think about such a thing. You'll never end up in there. Yes, you have a psychosis, as the doctor calls it, but you're not that ill. Besides, asylums don't even exist anymore. They're way in the past."

"*I don't have any psychosis! All that's wrong with me is my platelets are sticking.*"

So much for increasing awareness, I thought. How can she have such terrible fears one moment, obviously indicating that she knew that she had a mental illness, and then the next moment deny it altogether? I, in my role as an English teacher, had always enjoyed paradoxes, but this one ... I just couldn't seem to accept that such a paradox as this, this real and scary one regarding my own Kaija, could exist.

Nevertheless, I had to live with the day-to-day details of life, and since Kaija obviously was unable to handle even the simplest financial transactions, I decided that I'd better get a power of attorney so that I could look after these for both of us. We had always shared in these duties—she was a much better bookkeeper than me—and we had always had joint bank accounts. When I mentioned this to her, she readily agreed, and even showed relief, as if this were a burden she was glad to be rid of. When the time came to sign the papers, she commented to me, "It's good we're doing this because it will show that I'm sane."

It was hard for me to get a read on her, for these moments of seeming insight were always but flashes of light amongst days of continuing darkness. Nevertheless, they kept the flicker of hope alive in me and gave me renewed energy and resolve to bring her out of this inner world as often as I could.

Chapter 14: Compulsions and Obsessions

As always, it seemed to me that just as my hopes were mounting, a dash of cold water extinguished them. This time I was really frightened, for now Kaija began once more to act upon the messages she received. This had not happened for a long time, not since she had so many times packed her clothes to go *"to the new house"* when she had been home on her first passes last fall.

What happened became also the beginning of one of her first and endless obsessions: *"Jean Wallin, my first grade teacher, has deposited a hundred and fifty thousand dollars into our account,"* Kaija said as she dressed and put on her coat to go to the bank one day.

"You can't just walk there; it's too far for you," I answered.

"Well, we have to go there to sign a three-hundred-thousand-dollar bank draft."

"There is no bank draft, hon. Why would anyone send us that much money?"

"Because I was her favorite student in school."

I convinced her to take her coat off and managed to distract her by beginning to get lunch on the table. But the next morning, first thing: *"We'll be late getting to the bank. We we're supposed to be there at 9:00 AM to sign that draft. Let's go!"*

She went on and on about it. Finally I decided that the only way to overcome this one was to take her to the bank so she could hear from the teller that there was no bank draft. I made her ask the teller herself, even though it hurt me to expose her illness so openly to someone who had no knowledge of it. But she had to be satisfied and hear it from the horse's mouth, so I raised my eyebrow surreptitiously to signal the teller that my wife was having mental difficulties. Told that there was no bank draft, Kaija looked disappointed and confused, but did not press the issue.

The next day it was the same thing all over. She harassed me so many times to take her to sign the draft *"that's come in now"* that I finally gave in and took her there again. This time the loans manager gave her the same answer. Surely that will convince her, I thought. But it was not to be. Two days later it started all over again, only this time I resolutely refused to take her there. She cried, but soon got over it.

For a few days she seemed to have forgotten the issue, but then it burst forth again. When I again said I would not take her because it was Saturday, she replied, *"The supervisor is coming to get me."* As usual, though, when no action occurred, she forgot about it—for a day or two.

So obsessed did she become again within a few days that I once more gave in and took her to the bank. Before we went though, I phoned the bank manager and asked if they could have some kind of official-looking standard document that Kaija could sign. I knew she would not read it anyway, and maybe this would satisfy her that the money was in. No doing! She signed the fake document, all right, but we no sooner got home than Kaija said, *"We have to go back again. That was the wrong document."*

In exasperation, I took her back one more time. This time she was given just a signature card to sign and for the moment seemed satisfied. But at home, *"We need to go back because there's still a release form to sign."* I would not take her. Instead, I suggested I go alone and if there actually was such a form, I would bring it home for her to sign. I knew now that this could go on and on and that I would have to try something different.

The manager was glad to see me and invited me into her office. "This has got to stop," she said. "I can't have our tellers being disturbed and harassed this way."

"That's exactly why I'm here alone this time—to talk about it and to determine some new course of action to take my problem off your shoulders. It's not your responsibility. Can you suggest anything?"

"From now on we won't try to humor her, since that obviously did not work. If she comes in, or even calls, we'll firmly tell her that everything has been looked after, that there are no documents for her to sign, and that she shouldn't expect any."

"That's what I was thinking," I said. "We've got to stop this somehow or the charade could go on for months. We've been toying with it for over two weeks already. But if you would be so kind as to give me one more piece of paper for her to sign, I'll try my best to convince her that this is final. And I just won't bring her here anymore. Eventually, she'll have to get the message."

Kaija did not get the message. The next morning she dressed in her best black suit and pink blouse and three times insisted that we go to the bank. When I refused to take her, she went upstairs, miffed. I soon followed her and found her sitting on the bed, a blank look on her face. Had the message sunk in? I wondered. But no—at least five or six times that same afternoon she kept saying things like, *"There's an affidavit to sign … The exchange rate changed and we have to re-sign … My signature was no good because my hand shook … Did you know your Aunt Mary died? Her head exploded … They'll close our account if we don't get there today …"*

My exasperation knew no bounds, yet I managed to control my temper and firmly kept telling her that the bank draft was all taken care of. The matter came up intermittently over the next few weeks, but soon another obsession became overlaid on the first, and my energies were diverted to the new one.

"You have to go to the health food store and get me a bottle of Beef, Iron and Wine. I should have been on it long ago," Kaija said, in no uncertain terms one day.

"What are you talking about?" I asked. "I've never in all my life heard of such a thing."

"Well, if you haven't, I have! It's a drink that builds up red corpuscles and keeps your liver healthy. It gives you energy, besides. Whenever we were worn down after a flu, Grandma would get out this brown bottle and give us two or three ounces of it."

I was sure she had just dreamed this all up, that it was

just another hallucination. "I'll go to the health store and ask about it," I said to mollify her.

"I've never heard of such a drink," Christy, the clerk, said. "It sounds like a homemade recipe to me—you know, something the farmers of early days could mix up right at home. Let me check my catalogs, though ... No, I don't have that listed under any of my suppliers."

"I'm sure it's just one of Kaija's hallucinations anyway, but thanks for checking it out."

"I need to have Beef, Iron and Wine for my platelets," she insisted, many times a day, every day. It was beginning to drive me crazy. "If you can't get that, go to the store and ask the meat guy to give you some fresh beef liver. *My platelet count is so low now that I'll die soon because my liver will just dry out. It's only at forty-four and if it goes below forty, I'll die. Allan passed away tonight from the same thing. He died at the station. He didn't even get home. So I need that medicine."*

"OK, here's your liver, Kaija," I said after returning from my mission. "There's enough here for three meals. I even bought some onions for you to fry it in. That's how you like it, don't you?

"Yes. We used to eat it just after we got married, but I haven't made it for a long, long time since neither of us liked it very much."

"Yeah. Don't bother making any for me; I'll find something else to eat whenever you have that. Here, I went to the health food store and bought you some iron pills, too. Christy said these would be the best thing for your platelets. They should help build up your blood, too."

"*I know. The doctor just told me I'm to take three a day.*"

"Good heavens, you can't do that! You'll be so constipated within two days that you'll end up in the hospital. I wish you wouldn't listen to those doctors on 'ad lib.' They never, ever tell the truth. You've seen that a hundred times. I wish you'd trust Dr. McRae for once. You've been fighting to not take your Respiradol pills for two weeks now, yet that's the most important of all the meds you're on."

"*I said I'm not taking it anymore because it will kill me ... and you can't make me!*"

"So I've found out! Listen, Dr. McRae told you two days ago that your platelet count was normal, at 239. Look, it's right here on this sheet he gave me, listing all the blood test results. He said the normal range is between 150 and 450."

"*I don't care what that sheet says. My blood platelet count is forty-two over thirty-eight and those pills aren't doing me any good at all. You just want me to die by making me take them. When I do, just have them put on my gravestone, 'Her husband killed her with pills.'* And I'm not going back to Dr. McRae anymore either!"

So Kaija, self-diagnosed and self-administered, ate five meals of liver in a row before she got tired of it. If she dies now, they'll have to beat her liver to death with a stick, I thought. She likely would have taken the three iron pills a day, too, if I had let her, but since I gave her her pills every day, I let her have only one along with her other meds in the morning.

"*These iron pills are not what I need*" became the obsessive refrain again. "*I need to have Beef, Iron and Wine to get my red blood count up. It comes in a red ampoule, so go ask Christy to give you one. She's probably got some in by now."*

"I told you she doesn't even know what it is!"

I refused to go. Just to reassure myself (Kaija was so convincing!) that there was no such thing, I got on the Internet, Googled "Beef Iron and Wine" and was shocked to see two Web sites come up that listed exactly that! So she had been right. I should have known ... she had an elephant's memory, and this illness had certainly not affected that, I had discovered over and over these past few months.

Both sites were in the southwest states: Alabama and Tennessee. Quack stuff, I thought. No explanations about contents, no medical endorsements, no directions even on how much to take, or for what. Five dollars and ninety-five cents for a twenty-five-ounce bottle. Well, I'd order a bottle and at least get Kaija off my back about this issue. It likely couldn't do any harm, and I could monitor it carefully. The checkout basket brought me another surprise—shipping and handling: $24.95! Good heavens—four times the cost of the medicine! But that didn't deter me; anything I could do to get rid of Kaija's obsession would bring me some peace as well.

The bottle came two weeks later. I made a big thing of showing her the package, saying that more would be shipped later. There were no directions on the brown plastic bottle either, so I made up my own. The liquid was a very dark brown, so I figured I could dilute it and Kaija would never be the wiser. I bought eight cartons of Apple, Peach and Passion Fruit juice from the Co-op, took them home, mixed an ounce of Beef, Iron and Wine into each of countless pint jars of juice, and hid them in the basement. I put a half dozen into the fridge, thinking that I would just replace them daily as she used them up. It bothered me, though, to be pulling the wool over her eyes this way and constantly having to tell her white lies. This was not the sharp, intelligent lady I had married and lived with for the last forty years.

To my amazement, when I looked in the fridge after coming back from a shopping trip to the city the next day, there was not a single pint left!

"What did you do with that Beef, Iron and Wine I mixed for you? Did you throw it all out or what? There aren't even any empty jars around!"

"No. I didn't throw them out. I drank them all. *I'm supposed to drink six pints a day for the first three days and then cut back on it gradually to four cups a day.* I washed the jars and took them back into the basement."

"That 'ad lib' junk is telling you some gross lies again! Do you realize you're going to have really bad diarrhea from this? Nobody can drink that amount of juice in a day, day after day. The directions on the Internet said to take from eight to ten ounces a day maximum," I lied. "I guess I'll just have to mix you one pint a day and give it to you with your morning meds.

"Oh! You make me so mad! You treat me like a little child."

"Listen, hon, the doctor said that either Home Care or I am to administer your meds, and that's what we've been doing, or trying to do since you came home. We can't trust those 'ad lib' directions—they're all screwed up. So just trust me, OK?"

"Oh yeah, and you've been giving me Trazadone and I

was supposed to be off that two months ago! I don't need any antidepressants anymore."

"I'm not going to argue about it. The doctor hasn't said to stop Trazadone. You can have a pint of that Beef Iron stuff a day. Even that's way over the recommended limit of eight to ten ounces a day."

And so Kaija took her Beef, Iron and Wine religiously for five weeks. I began to panic, because the juice mix was getting low. What would I do then? I sure wasn't going to order that stuff again. Ah! Soy sauce, I thought. That's dark, too, but with just a bit of it in each jar, she'll never know the difference.

She did know! "This is Rilla, isn't it?" she asked when she tasted the first glassful.

"Rilla?" I asked.

"Yes. That's supposed to replace the Beef, Iron and Wine after five or six weeks. They sell it at the Co-op. It's mixed into apple and orange juice so it doesn't taste bad. You can get some after you go to Marv's memorial service. I can't go. I'm so weak because my platelets are still low, but you'd better go since he's your brother."

Marv, my brother, had certainly not died, but I had learned by now that it was best not to respond to such hallucinations and just to ignore them. Denying their truth was hopeless because to Kaija they were as real as real could be. Hallucinations about death had been especially prominent since she had come home. Once when I had come home from visiting Kaija's father in Home Care, she had been all dressed up in her dress suit and was boiling a pot of coffee on the stove. "How come you're making a full pot at this time of day?" I asked.

"*Because Esther and Walter and Lars and Lillian and a bunch of others are coming over because you died.*"

"Hon, I'm standing right here before you; I can't have died."

"*Yes, you did, but your other self came back. Did you get some more Rilla? I'm all out because I drank the three pints you had in the fridge.*"

"Yes, I got some." This was at least the twentieth time, the twentieth day (not consecutive) that she had hounded me about Rilla. I was getting weary from it all, and tired of having to mix the drink in secret all the time in the basement. Once she told me that there were four gallons of it ready-mixed at the health food store. If only it were that easy, I thought. This business of mixing in soy to darken the "Rilla" to give it a somewhat bitter taste was not so easy. The soy always separated into little globs and I had to shake it hard for a couple of minutes each time in order to get it to dissolve entirely. I immediately felt the familiar guilt pangs over my internal grumbling; this was the least I could do for her, and though it wasn't making her better, at least it relieved her anxiety and satisfied one of her overriding obsessions. And gave me some small measure of peace!

I needed that, I was beginning to believe. I needed relief from the growing stress. The health nurses were always preaching at me, "You have to look after yourself, too. You'll be of no help to your wife if you become burned out."

At first I had been somewhat angry at them for even suggesting such a thing. "Look, I'm strong and healthy. Just because I'm on antidepressants doesn't mean I can't cope. We're talking about Kaija here, not me." But as time went on and the obsessions not only continued but mounted in frequency and intensity, I had begun to think that perhaps they were right. But I fought against it. I would do anything for Kaija, and this did not, in my mind, include pampering myself. That was why I had taken the semester leave from teaching, after all.

But then again, had I not already partially shifted the focus to myself? Already by the end of January I felt myself slipping. Things were getting to me, in spite of my early resolve to accept whatever Kaija's homecoming would bring. I had purposely gone for long walks, indulged in more sweets than normal, escaped into easy-reading Western novels whenever possible. But none of these things had any lasting benefit. They kept me sane (what irony, I thought, applying that word to myself). Yet that thought had been the one that drove me to seek psychiatric help for myself.

I had long ago shed any stigma I had had about mental illness. I had not been immune to the common thoughts and responses of the general public toward those who were "off the beam," just another of the common phrases used to describe any abnormal behavior in an individual. I had known more than one individual—even one relative—who had some form of psychosis or other. I had related to them just fine, had even enjoyed chatting with them from time to time and felt that I treated them as equals. Yet when I was with others, I was just as apt as they to talk about the individual who was "one brick short of a load," had "one cog missing," was "crazy as a coot," was "off his rocker." The list of degrading idioms went on and on. I felt ashamed that I had so thoughtlessly used them.

Although Kaija's psychiatrist had put me on Lorazepam, a common mood-leveling medication, late last fall while Kaija was still in the Elliston Unit, I felt that I needed something more. So I made an appointment with a different psychiatrist, hoping for I knew not what. Maybe just an outsider's understanding of my situation, maybe some advice on how to respond to Kaija or to help her, maybe for reassurance that I, myself, was doing OK, or maybe just for some kind of miracle.

Dr. Khan was objectively empathetic. He listened. He understood. He asked relevant questions and sought to know the reasons for my worries and fears. And so began a series of meetings in which Dr. Khan applied cognitive therapy—a treatment that I had heard of but had never known what it actually meant.

It involved a lot of talking and discussion about me and my life situation, both past and present. These Dr. Khan picked up on, and taught me to consider and evaluate the positive aspects of each experience, each year, of my and Kaija's shared life, and each bump in the road of the present situation that made life a challenge for me.

I was glad I went to Dr. Khan. It was different unloading to a stranger, but more importantly, to a professional who understood and knew how to help me. As Kaija's obsessions and compulsive behaviors escalated, I needed all the help I could get.

At the beginning of March Kaija absolutely refused to take her Respiradol pills. The Home Care nurses had had to cajole her every time for the past three weeks into letting them give the shot, and sometimes it took a full ten minutes to succeed. Each time she put up more resistance.

Finally, at the beginning of March she adamantly refused. There was nothing the nurses or I could do.

Fortunately, Kaija had an appointment with Dr. McRae the following week. At the appointment she complained, as always, of her platelet count being low. Dr. McRae showed her the true number again, but Kaija's response was, *"Those are not my results; they're for someone else."*

"We'll just give you a 'tonic' then. I can see that you need something to pick you up."

And so, "Rilla" eventually gave way to a "tonic." Although Kaija didn't know it, the tonic was Respiradol in liquid form. Kaija didn't even ask to see the bottle. She knew that the prescription was for two milligrams per day, but she made up her own recipe for it: *"Two milligrams of tonic in two teaspoons of honey and one tablespoon of cognac, in a quarter glass of water."* I substituted cooking wine for the cognac, and she took the medicine willingly. I had provided her with Beef, Iron and Wine, and "Rilla," and so she trusted me to also do the same with the tonic. I was relieved. At least I didn't have to continue making pint upon pint of "medicine" for her anymore.

The tonic seemed to make Kaija accept her meds without argument for a while, but it did nothing to reduce her obsessions.

"We've got to send our whole set of Cutco knives to New York to get sharpened. They told me yesterday on 'ad lib.'" "Well, yes, some of them should be sharpened," I agreed. We've had them for twenty-one years now so it's no wonder if some of them are dull."

"And the paring knife should be replaced because the

tip is broken on it. *It just fell off one day when I was cutting an apple.*"

"It's been broken for a long time, hon. I broke it when I was prying a lid off a jar one day."

"Well, whatever."

That was the introduction to a new harassment that lasted over many weeks. I could have shortened it if I had been on the bit and just agreed to send the knives in right away. However, I couldn't remember what kind of warranty they had, or where, for sure, to ship them. Nor did I think I should send in the complete set, so I put off doing anything about the knives and tried a diversion tactic instead.

One day, probably in late March, I came home from the city with a six-week-old, jet black little poodle in my arms. I knew that people sometimes brought their little dogs into the Riverview Care Home where Kaija's dad lived, just to cheer up the elderly patients (all level five) that lived there and to bring a bit of diversion into their lives. I had read, too, that having a pet was often therapeutic for people with anxiety problems, high stress levels, or burnout.

Years ago, soon after Kaija had her surgery for breast cancer, I did the same thing, the same way—by surprise. I would never forget the joy on Kaija's face when I set the little pooch on the floor and it had immediately waddled right up to her. She picked it up in her arms, hugged it, let it lick her face, and laughed and cried at the same time. From that moment on, Misty became her dog, her best friend. It brought her immeasurable comfort and delight over the next six months of chemotherapy. She taught it to lie at the foot of the bed and they became inseparable companions.

But I was disappointed. Kaija's reaction to the pup was lukewarm at best. Oh, she picked it up and held it and let it nuzzle her, but she soon turned it over to me.

"He's so cute and lovable, but he's too heavy and rambunctious for me. You'd better take him now."

"OK. I'll set up the training cage and then you can feed him. Would that be all right?" I wanted to get her actively involved so that she would have some real life focus. Alas, it was not to be.

"Did you mail those Cutco knives in when you went to the city?" she asked, while pouring the dry dog food into Trixie's dish.

"No, I didn't," I said, completely deflated. My attempt had fallen flat. Kaija seemed to like Trixie fine, but she had other concerns weighing on her mind.

"*I got the address from one of the managers on 'ad lib' today.*" Sure enough, she handed me a sticky note with an address painfully written in her shaky handwriting:

Cutco Knives, Inc.
1535 E. Cumberland Cutco Knives Inc.
New York, NY 20028
USA

Below was a note: "Insure each knife for two hundred dollars."

It looked so authentic that I was almost inclined to believe that it was correct. Since this obsession was over-ruling everything else, including Trixie, I decided I'd better try something to appease her. I had a belated brain wave: check the Internet for the address. Of course

I found it immediately, but it was far different from the one Kaija had given me. And there was a Canadian address, too.

"They have to go back to New York," Kaija insisted when I told her. *"The guy there knows us; he said to send in our complete set and they would just exchange it for a new one. Even Trixie says that's what we should do. She talks to me all the time.* And I want them to give us a black set instead of the white one we have now.'

"Well, I don't think they'll do that but I'll phone them to find out." Indeed, Kaija knew, or remembered, much better than me, as usual. The knives had come with a lifetime guarantee, and the salesman I talked to said yes, they would exchange the whole set and we could have a black-handled set in place of the white.

I wrapped up the set and mailed it the next day. I didn't let Kaija see the Canadian address, though.

Three weeks and twenty or more annoying references to the new, black-handled knives coming from New York passed before they finally did arrive—from Ontario. Kaija saw the return address and wouldn't even open the package. All the excitement that I had anticipated from her did not materialize.

"These aren't our knives. Send them back and tell them that our set is in New York."

"They are so ours. I mailed our old set to the Ontario branch because that's where the guy on the phone told me to send them. All Canadian orders go there. Let's just open the box, OK, so that you can see what's in it."

"You go ahead. I don't want to see them. Neither does Trixie. Dogs can smell the right thing, you know."

So I opened the package, and yes, there was a full

set of knives with black handles, each one protected in an individual plastic case. This was exactly what Kaija wanted, but was unwilling to accept *"because they're not ours."* I took all of the knives out of their cases, and put them into their butcher-block holder. Kaija would have to face the reality of them being there and see me using them daily; perhaps she would gradually lose her obsession about where they came from and whose they were.

That's exactly what happened. Trixie was largely responsible for that. After four or five weeks I gave the pup to Kaija's nephew, Matt and his family. Kaija had mostly ignored it, and certainly had taken no part in looking after it. I had loved playing with it, but training it and looking after it had become a bit much. Kaija agreed to giving her away, and I thought that was the end of that.

I didn't realize, however, that through "ad lib" Kaija had forged a close relationship with Trixie. *"Trixie and I still talk all the time,"* she told me. *"It's just the same as having her here."*

So that's why she didn't really care about the knives, I thought. Her mind was fixated on something else now. One day she told me an incredible story: *"Funny how that cat, Troy, was there at Matt and Katie's, and Trixie asked her if she was a believer—'cause Trixie understands cat language – and Troy said he wasn't because he came from a family that never went to church and they had never taught him about faith. So then Trixie blessed him and then they both asked me to bless them. So I did, and then they blessed me."*

Truth—even truth of the inner mind—was surely stranger than fiction, I thought again as I listened to her story. As sad as my wife's condition was, the story made me laugh. Kaija didn't mind my laughter, for she was so happy about the story that she laughed in joy at *"how well Troy and Trixie got along."*

This ability to talk with animals didn't really surprise me, for often when the geese were flying overhead to settle on the nearby river for the night, Kaija had smiled and made such comments as, *"The geese are talking to me"* and *"The geese tell me all kinds of things because they can see so far when they fly up high."* They obviously had a good relationship, too, for though Kaija never told me what the geese said, she was always smiling when she told me about them.

The hallucinations and delusions about Trixie came to an end rather abruptly: *"Troy, that cat, peed on Trixie's blanket so now she won't play with it. Matt and Katie are going to have to get rid of Trixie because she is so unhappy ... Oh! Matt just took Trixie out to the caragana hedge and shot her."*

Never again did she mention Trixie. And she began to use her new Cutco knives about this time, too!

One thing that I found trying was the nightly ritual in the bathroom when getting ready for bed. It wasn't that it bothered my nerves for I had learned to hear Kaija talking aloud on "ad lib" many times a day. I asked her a number of times whom she was talking to, and if it was a happy conversation, she would sometimes tell me. But the negative ones she mostly kept to herself. Kaija continued to lock me out, and I was left to conjecture, based on what I heard her say.

The reason I had such a hard time with the bathroom conversations this time was that they were always of such a tormenting nature. It was classic paranoia, and I just felt so sorry for her, having to suffer so. She would be very angry, and would speak at full voice behind the locked bathroom door. The light was always off, too. Regular lockdown procedure, I thought. A couple of times I had knocked on the door to try to calm her down and to console her, and although she opened the door to me, she remained in a high stage of agitation. The episodes would usually last from ten to fifteen minutes. There was always a lot of repetition of some phrases, the most common ones being *"Shut up! Leave me alone! Why don't you get lost!"*

There was always more—much more—full-fledged, one-sided (to my ears) conversations (or yelling matches, to be more accurate). Each night there were variations in the content, but always they were loud and angry. My helplessness was magnified during these times, but because the conversations were a nightly ritual, I eventually learned to block them out. No doubt I was, unconsciously, protecting my own sanity in doing so.

It was the repetition of so many, many issues that wore me down. The bathroom scenes were only one of the hundreds of repeated (with some variations) comments and demands that I heard over a period of five months. I learned that to distract her, or to simply agree to them, was best. She'd soon forget them, at least for a little while. To oppose her was the worst thing I could do, for it inevitably brought about a confrontation and escalation in frustration, anxiety, and anger.

The demands were the hardest to deal with and they were there daily: *"Let's go to the new house ... Get me some boxes so I can start packing ... Take me to the bank ... Dr. Naipaul is waiting for us at the house; let's go already,"* and on and on. Of course I could never fulfill her wishes (I had tried once with the bank issue) and this both frustrated me and wore me down. It came to the point where I needed to get away for a while, to focus on my own health and state of mind. When my sister and one of her daughters decided to make a trip to Minnesota to visit other family members, I used this as my reason for getting away for a few days and hopped in their ride. I got Kaija's sister, Esther, to stay with her.

"Do you really mean you're going to go?" she asked one day.

I had told her of my plans earlier, a few days back, and had repeated them a couple more times, hoping that she would get used to the idea. But now, as the day for my departure was imminent, she was devastated.

"You mean you're actually going to go and leave me here all alone?"

"No, hon, you won't be alone. I've arranged for Esther to come and stay with you for the whole time I'm gone."

"You don't even care, do you? You don't even care if I die! Lots of people die when they're left alone. Anyway, you can't go because your sister is in hell."

"None of that is true, hon, and you know it. You know I love you. It's just that I need a bit of a break from the everyday routine. I know you do, too, and if you were well enough, of course we'd go together. I'll only be gone five days, and I'll phone you every evening, OK?"

And so I went, leaving my Kaija behind in tears. All had gone fairly well, but she chose this time to refuse to take another of her medications—Wellbutrin, her antidepressant. *"They're off the market because people have died from them"* was the familiar refrain. I wondered if my being away had anything to do with it, but there was no way to know. When she had gone off her Respiradol shots, I had been home, and then, as now, her refusal was absolute and adamant. I phoned her in the evenings, but she was flat and had nothing to say. I also talked with Esther, and learned that the first day Kaija said there were four of me, but Esther couldn't see them because we were invisible. On each day following, she insisted that I was dead.

"How come you're here?" she asked me when I got home. *"You're not supposed to be here. You died a few days ago."*

"No, hon, I'm alive and right here with you."

But where was Kaija, my own beloved? It was not her who stood before me. Mockingly, I heard in my mind Dylan Thomas' poetic words: "Though lovers be lost love shall not / And death shall have no dominion." Love I had in abundance, but my own true love was, indeed, lost. But I clung to the last line. My death persona, so alive in Kaija's mind, would not get me—neither I, nor God, would allow it!

Kaija said no more but just looked at me as though she was looking right through me at something, or someone, beyond. After supper she said, *"You'd better go quickly because Taivaan Valtion Isa is calling to you from heaven."*

Death was perhaps the most insidious of all her obsessions. She had such hallucinations many times before, but right from the time she came home from the hospital they seemed almost to possess her. As April turned into May, and May into June, they increased in frequency (almost daily now), and whereas before they mostly involved me, or close family members, the obsession now expanded to include whomever happened to pop into her mind, or more correctly, to invade her "ad lib." I was intrigued by this, for it showed how widely her inner mind ranged even though her daily real-life focus was so narrow—on herself, mostly. On April Fools' Day (the irony did not escape me) I began to record many of the death episodes that surfaced from her spoken thoughts: *"Alfred passed away at four o'clock today. He died at the railway station ... Marv's memorial is tonight. You have to go to it since he's your brother. I can't go because I need to rest, but it's imperative that you go. Don't forget to take flowers ... Aunt Mary died today; she fell on her head. Robert was there when it happened and he said she died right away ... You have to go to Marv's funeral, too, not just the memorial* (this four days in a row) *... Arnold passed away while he was just sitting in a chair. He just slept away. That's another one from that generation gone ... All four Stevenson boys just died—Ben, Ryan, Don, and Trent ... You died yesterday. Your funeral will be on Friday. I probably won't get there because of my platelets ... I'm going back upstairs because the other Arnold is there, the one who didn't get into heaven. But the other one did. I'm going to make supper for him so that he won't die, too ... I thought you had died; how come you're here? Oh, it was Mo, your other you, who died ... Taivaan Valtion Isa is dying; I won't be able to talk to him anymore ... He and Jesus are waiting to take you to heaven so that they can fibrillate your heart ... Laestadius told me to quit smoking because he's going to preach—oh, he just passed away ... The heavenly Father and Lord Jesus are waiting for you at the back door. Get going! They've been* *waiting for fifteen minutes already ... I have blank spells for twenty minutes to a half hour. I just black out so I'll die soon if I don't get that drink ... I'll die of mitral stenosis if I don't smoke six cigarettes a day ... Don't be so smart. You think you know everything. I wish you'd just drop dead ... Helvi Jones just died of a massive hemorrhage. I was just talking with Drew and he is sad. She was so young ... I'm not taking those pills; all you want is for me to die* (for the hundredth time!) ... "

From the beginning Kaija balked at taking many of her prescribed medications. Although it frustrated me, I could understand her reaction, for she had had more med changes in the past year than I had in my lifetime. At the end of March she was put on the Wellbutrin for her depression. Citalopram was to be reduced gradually. I didn't even know when she started on that one, or which doctor had prescribed it; there were just too many for me to keep up with. I wondered why they were now focusing on the depression instead of the psychosis, but then, I recalled, the label they had given her when all this first started: "psychotic depression." So perhaps it made sense after all.

What began to bother me was that physically Kaija had changed so much over the past few months. She was always tired. Was it from side effects of the medications, or a natural part of depression, or something else? The something else bothered me because it seemed to me that since the focus was on the psychosis, and rightly so, Kaija's physical health was not monitored as closely as it should have been—at least in my mind. I discovered that she lost three more pounds in the past two weeks. That made a total of twenty four pounds altogether. She was so skinny and frail that she walked with a shuffle, and very slowly and carefully. Her shoulders were hunched forward, her head down. She looked eighty years old, and seemed to be just withering away.

Both Dr. Liu and Dr. McRae told me that weight loss was a common occurrence with depression. I knew that, but it seemed to me that Kaija's was excessive—she looked anorexic. I was afraid that she was on the road to an early death. Perhaps Kaija felt this, too, and that was what drove her death delusions. I was just guessing; I always tried to find a logical explanation for everything that took place. Stupid of me, I thought. How can the rational be applied to the irrational? I wanted answers, but to date, all answers to all of my questions had been tentative and too general to mean much.

I read and read. I researched every drug as soon as she was given it. I learned the range of dosages for different conditions (not that I could keep them all in my head), and what symptom(s) each one was treating. Even that was crazy. So far the medical professionals had been treating symptoms, not the specific illness. They readily acknowledged that, for they still did not know what had brought the psychosis on, nor did they know what exactly they were treating. Psychotic depression was just a label to make discussion of the illness easier. They preferred to just say that Kaija was living with a psychosis.

And so I read and read about different psychoses: schizophrenia, bipolar disorder, anorexia, bulimia, and paranoia. I, too, focused mainly on the symptoms of each. Symptoms were easy to see and, therefore, understand. From Google I downloaded the document, "Out of the Shadows at Last," a two-and-a-half-year study on mental health commissioned by the federal government. I read every word of it, but all the knowledge in the world would not help me to really understand or accept Kaija's illness. I needed to get inside her head, just as I had gotten inside her heart over our lifetime together. I could read her emotions as though they were spelled out on paper.

But I could not read her mind. Before, I was sometimes able to, but not anymore. A different mind was housed within her now, not the mind of my wife. I remembered the doctor's diagnosis of Lady Macbeth: "She is troubled with thick coming fancies / that keep her from her rest." So true, so true of my own Kaija, I thought. And I identified fully with Macbeth when in exasperation he had replied, "Cure her of that. Canst not minister to a mind diseased?"

I ached to be able to help her, but there was really nothing of any significance that I could do. I would just have to keep on loving her and giving from my heart what I could not give from my head.

Chapter 15: Crisis

Things came to a head rather quickly in June. Just as Kaija's obsessions had increased in frequency and intensity, so had her hallucinations and her antagonism toward her medications. I could not get over how varied, strange, and bizarre her delusions and hallucinations could be. The bathroom scenes ratcheted up many notches. I recorded one of them: *"I'm not brushing my teeth tonight ... I said I'm not brushing my teeth tonight ... And I'm not showering in the morning because we're moving ... I will not take my watch off ... I hate this time of night so badly, with everyone yapping at me all the time ... Oh, you're such a lady, you know everything. I don't have to listen to you ... Shut your mouth. I don't want to hear one word from you. Shut your mouth, I said ... I get screamed at all day long. No one else does ... I'm talking about this channel we're on ... Who's talking? You don't know anything you're talking about ... Shut your mouth, you stupid ass. I'm never talking to my family again, or letting any of you into my house ... Quit poking my leg. Why do you always have to torment me?"*

After Kaija was home for about five months, I thought I had heard all the hallucinations possible. How mistaken and shortsighted this thought proved to be. No doubt one factor was that she went off two of her most important meds, but no matter how I or the Home Care nurses tried to encourage, cajole, or insist, she continued to refuse to take them.

One day near the end of May, Kaija decided she should reduce her tonic to one milligram instead of two, and to take it only every second night. The "recipe" for the tonic of a tablespoon of cognac and one of honey to a glass of water had been her own, so I was extremely disappointed that even Kaija's own prescriptions were now in jeopardy. So the Respiradol was now reduced to one quarter of what it should have been. I couldn't think of any other tricks I could use to get the antipsychotics into her, nor could Dr. McRae come up with anything. We discussed disguising it in coffee or juice, but we discarded that idea because the Respiradol was too bitter and Kaija would notice at once.

The hallucinations and obsessions immediately increased fivefold, and when a week later she stopped the Respiradol altogether, her temperament went quickly from bad to worse. She was restless, anxious, paranoid, and angry. Most of the hallucinations were reincarnations of the earlier ones, and she harassed me daily about going to the new house, going to the bank, and going to one funeral or another, most often my own. For some reason, she began to "communicate" a lot in Finnish. Perhaps she regressed within the confines of her psychotic mind, for Finnish was her first language as a child, and many of the "ad lib" conversations and laments were with family members and about bodily functions that were part of childhood learning.

"Who phoned?" she asked in anger one day. I was taken aback by the anger for I could see no cause for it unless the ringing of the phone had disturbed her "ad lib."

"Your sister called just to see how you're feeling."

"I suppose again she's phoning from hell."

Well, maybe that explains her anger, I thought. Likely Kaija didn't want me to be in contact with those in hell, especially when she so often told me that I had died and gone to heaven, or that God and Jesus were waiting for me at the door. But then, this was mere speculation, speculation from my rational mind, I reminded myself, and nothing was rational in her psychotic state. It was useless for me to try to explain Kaija's statements or behavior from my perspective. Once again I felt like Macbeth, who lamented that "My thought ... is so smothered in surmise, and nothing is / But what is not."

In Finnish she lashed out one day from the quiet of her bedroom, *"I'm sitting on my own side of the bed! He sleeps on the other side. Your nature is such that I could just kick you sometimes."* A little later she complained bitterly, still in Finnish, *"You don't let me do anything. I can't even set my foot on the floor or rise from my bed ... What's it to you if Kaija has to pee in her pants and lie in a wet bed? Some sister you are!"*

Another day her whole family was the object of her wrath: *"You're all ridiculing me the whole time so that I don't even want to live anymore."* Then she singled out her brother, Lars, as she often did: *"You're such a shithead I could just shoot you! Go lie in your own poop!"*

It was Lars, too, who was the "cause" of her somatic hallucinations. Always, it was *"He's poking me."*

"Where does he poke you?" I asked.

"Everywhere. Sometimes my knee or my hip, sometimes my back, everywhere—my stomach, my neck, my forehead. I can't get away from him. The only way I can is to make a tent with my quilt and hide under it. Sometimes he can't get me in the basement when I go for a smoke."

"Did he bug you a lot when you were kids? Did he always poke you, or touch you?" It was a loaded question, implying that perhaps Lars had verbally or even physically abused her when they were kids. But in all sincerity, Kaija replied, *"No. He only started after this business started. Anyway, it's the "other" Lars that does it."*

"What do you mean—what business?"

"Ever since all this 'ad lib' started."

"Does it help if I'm with you?"

"Yes, sometimes he can't get at me then." But even as she said it, she cried out, *"Now he's at my ankle!"* At other times it was her wrist or arm or any spot on her body. So I wasn't as good a protector as I wished. Nevertheless, at times like this I would gently massage whichever spot this alter ego Lars was poking to try to ease her pain and ward off her attacker. I was pretty sure that the poking was really her way of explaining real pain—her fibromyalgia, or a headache, or indigestion after a meal. Of course I was rationalizing an irrational situation again.

It was inevitable. Now that Kaija was off her entire menu of medications, she deteriorated rapidly. She stayed in her bedroom all the time, lights off, blinds drawn, quilt up to her chin. From there I could hear "ad lib" conversations and shouting matches all throughout the day. In desperation, I phoned City Hospital and managed to arrange an emergency appointment with a psychiatrist on call, a Dr. Ahmed. I had a terrible fight to get Kaija there but I finally enticed her by explaining to her that the meds she had been on were obviously doing nothing for her platelets, so we needed to see a different doctor to change prescriptions. To this she agreed and finally consented to go.

I liked Dr. Ahmed. He was not old, but much older than Dr. Lewis, and I sensed within a few minutes that here was a man of much experience. He was very direct, asked Kaija real-life questions—not the stock ones that had always been asked before—and had a warm and winning way about him that brought out the best in Kaija. "I like him," she told me later.

Dr. Ahmed fulfilled my tongue-in-cheek prophesy. He did put Kaija on different medications: Lamotrigine and Zyprexa.

"Lamotrigine is a mood stabilizer," he said. "It sounds to me that you are angry a lot, and maybe you have reason to be with all those people bothering you on 'ad lib.' But it's no good if you're angry at them and no good if then you get angry with Charles and keep demanding that he do things he can't do. This medication is fast-acting and will make you feel better in a day or two."

I was a bit put out. "I can understand the Lamotrigine, but why are you starting her on Zyprexa again? Dr. Lewis had her on this earlier and it didn't do a lick of good. The only drug that has helped at all was Seroquel. She was put on it last summer right after she came to City Hospital, and it's the only time I've seen any measurable improvement. But for some reason Dr. Lewis changed her to Zyprexa after only three or four weeks."

"Yes, that's what her chart shows, but she was on that for only about five weeks before she began the ECT treatments. That's not really long enough to see if it's going to work or not. Sometimes it takes up to six months before a positive effect of an antipsychotic is evident. Besides, I still think Zyprexa is a better option for Kaija, and Zyprexa is faster-acting, too."

"Like, how fast?"

"I think we need to keep her on it for a minimum of five months."

"You mean to tell me she'll be in here for that long again?"

"I didn't say we have to admit her. I know you're in a difficult situation at home, but Kaija can take both medications there, as long as you give them to her to see that she gets them regularly. The Lamotrigine should kick in soon and that will make your daily living easier until the Zyprexa begins to work."

"OK. I have to trust your judgment. I just hope we're on the right track this time."

That had been on June 10. For two days Kaija had taken the meds and then decided that they, too, were off the market. On June 17 she was again admitted to the Elliston Wing.

Chapter 16: We've Been Here Before

I checked my journal. It was May 20 when Kaija first threw me for a loop by talking nonsense, as I then thought of it, and May 21 when she was admitted to Riverview Hospital. Just three days short of a year it all began! What a long, long year it had been. You would think, I thought, that a year so packed with happenings would go by quickly. The teaching part of it in the fall semester actually flew by, but after that, the six months when Kaija was at home seemed like an eternity. As I reflected on those past six months I wasn't surprised. Two things contributed to the dragging of time: the constant, never-ending repetition of hallucinations, paranoia, and obsessions, and my daily anticipation that today, or next week, Kaija would be better and life would return to normal.

Normal. What did that mean anymore? A vague, almost useless term. A cruel joke! Kaija had been normal for a psychotic depressive or a schizophrenic person for the past year. That in itself was a revelation to me: how vastly my thinking and understanding had changed over that time. How vastly Kaija's and my life had changed. How uncertain, how dramatically changed my expectations about the future had become. I knew now that my former distorted concept of normal was gone forever. The psychiatrists' warnings, the reading I had done about psychotic illnesses, and my own yearlong observations of Kaija's behavior convinced me that she would never return to normal as I had previously, unconsciously, conceived of it.

Now year two had begun with as much trauma as had year one. Once again I had to scramble, with the help of the district mental health nurse, Glenda McKenzie, to get a Form 18 signed by Dr. McRae and Dr. Ahmed so that I could take Kaija to the hospital against her will. Once again I had to create an exciting scene for the neighbors to gossip about. Once again I had to call the police and the ambulance to force my most beloved spouse to leave her home, to leave me, and to be admitted to the Dungeon. And once again we had to undergo a five-hour torture session in the ER before she was admitted.

Now-familiar patterns re-emerged: interviews by two unfamiliar psychiatrists, legal forms to be filled, a depressing hospital ward with locked doors in the Elliston Wing, sedatives, forced injections of antipsychotics, tears, and more tears.

In an ironic reversal, it was my turn to receive a new medication. When Kaija and I met with the psychiatrist the next morning, Dr. Ahmed took a long look at me. "You're living on the emotional edge, I can plainly see. You're trying to be strong for Kaija, but those tears just don't want to stop, do they?"

"I'm sorry. I feel like a schmo, crying and drawing attention to me. It's Kaija who needs your help."

"That's true, of course. But I can see that you need some help, too. We can't have you both ill at the same time. I'm going to prescribe you some Lamotrigine to help stabilize you. You won't necessarily have to be on it for a long time, but we'll try it and see how you do. Are you on any other medication?"

"Yes, I've been on antidepressants for the past two years. I've tried to go off them more than once because I didn't think I really needed them anymore. But every time I stopped them, especially this past year, I got so that I couldn't function properly. I was on Effexor for a long time, and once before, long ago when Kaija had cancer I was on Pamelor. But both of these caused me to ache, so right now Dr. McRae has me on three hundred milligrams of Wellbutrin twice a day."

"That's a pretty high dosage, and I don't think your trouble is as much depression as it is anxiety and stress. I'm going to change your Wellbutrin to one hundred fifty milligrams twice a day, and I want you to take one hundred milligrams of Lamotrigine morning and evening. I'll see you again in a month to see how you're doing."

"OK. But what about Kaija? It seems she's been on every antipsychotic there is, and here we are, still at step one. Even when she was still taking her Zyprexa, it didn't do her any good."

"I know that, but it's been only a few weeks since we stopped the Respiradol and started the Zyprexa. That's not a fair enough trial and I still think it's the best option. However, I'm going to try one other thing. I'm going to put her on a low dosage of another antipsychotic, Zydis, at the same time. Sometimes combinations have worked with patients who don't respond to a single antipsychotic, although the literature says that there is no evidence to support the use of more than one antipsychotic at a time. We don't like to do that until we've exhausted other possibilities, because then it is hard to measure which drug is having a positive effect, or sometimes which is causing a certain side effect. But we'll try this and monitor it closely. She needs to stay on Lamotrigine as well."

"How long will she have to be in this dark, dingy and crowded downstairs ward?"

"I don't know that. Although she's extremely agitated right now, I don't think she'll try to get away. It depends on when a bed becomes available upstairs. But I would suggest that you don't come to visit her for a week to ten days. She needs to settle in again, and if you come to see her, she will just expect every time that she can go home. This is too hard on the both of you and does not help Kaija at all right now."

Dr. Ahmed seemed to have summed up the situation well. As hard as it was on me to stay away, I nevertheless did so. I called and talked to the nurses every second day. They told me that Kaija was not cooperating in taking her meds, that she was often angry, agitated, and in tears, that she thought that I was waiting in the parking lot every day to take her home. *"He's invisible,"* she kept telling them when they refuted her.

I finally dared to talk to Kaija on the phone after two weeks had passed. The nurses told me that she had stabilized, that she was much more pleasant than when she was admitted, but that she stayed in her room except at meal times. When I called the first time and asked how she was, Kaija said she was "confused" but that she was "starting to get better." That was a big step—the admission that something was wrong, other than her platelets.

The next time I called, Kaija was quiet and subdued as before, but sounded, and even said that she was really happy that I had called. I was heartened by this simple expression of emotion—the first positive one I had heard in a long time. But what absolutely amazed me was her answer when I asked how she was feeling: "Oh, my mind isn't right; *I get confused and forget what people say on 'ad lib.' Sometimes I get blank spots so I can't even hear them.*"

The first part of the statement showed the clearest recognition that something was wrong mentally. And although the second part returned her to the fantasy world of "ad lib," it made me wonder if the voices were beginning to diminish in frequency and intensity. Could it be possible that they would some day fade away altogether? I hoped so.

I soon had another reason to hope. Soon after Kaija was readmitted, they ran an MRI. I didn't even know they were going to do an MRI, but I was pleased to hear that they had. MRIs, I knew, were relatively new; there were only two in the city. They developed out of, but were far superior to, CT scans (computerized tomography), which Kaija had right at the onset of her illness, even before she was admitted to City Hospital. From what I understood, magnetic resonance imaging was a superior way to gather microscopic chemical and physical information about molecules, in this case, in the brain. Although nuclear MRIs have been in initial stages of development since the early 1970s, the latest ones, in operation only since 2003, can map regions of the brain for thought and motor control. The test, therefore, made sense to me, as both the family doctors and the psychiatrists had explained that Kaija's psychosis was likely due to a chemical imbalance in the brain. If so, perhaps this test should help them determine whether or not there actually was a chemical imbalance, and indicate what had gone haywire with Kaija's thought control.

The good news was that the MRI had not shown any sign of brain abnormality. Or was it good news? Maybe some kinds of abnormalities were easier to fix than whatever Kaija's problem was.

Dr. Ahmed was rather vague in describing the results, perhaps because they were of a nature that only medical professionals would understand. In any case, after the test he did leave a shadow in my mind by saying, "It could be that Kaija will never recover full brain function." It must have been something in the MRI that led him to that observation, although Dr. Ahmed did not directly say so.

My meeting with Dr. Ahmed, in which I was informed of these events, occurred eighteen days after Kaija was admitted. I had not seen her in all this time and was a little apprehensive about going to see her even now. But the test results and Kaija's gradual improvements in compliance and disposition led Dr. Ahmed to suggest that it was time again to "test the waters" by giving Kaija a three-day pass home. I was surprised. It's too soon, I thought. In my mind there flashed only negative memories and images. I wasn't yet ready to face again such experiences as I had lived through in the past six months. I didn't believe that the Zydis/Zyprexa combination could have worked wonders in less than three weeks. I expressed my doubts to Dr. Ahmed, but was assured that this was "a necessary trial to see whether Kaija's behavior will remain as stable in her home environment as it has become here in a hospital setting."

And so, Kaija came home.

Disaster! I was befuddled. Why, oh why, was Kaija like this as soon as she walked in the door of her own home? Yes, she had been agitated, angry, obsessed, and delusional when she was readmitted to the Elliston Unit three weeks ago, but she had improved so much, according to the nurses and Dr. Ahmed. She had been pleasant, compliant, peaceful. But now it was just as if she had never been away, a repeat of her prehospital behavior.

"Are you going to get me some Jim Bream now?"

"Jim Bream? What's that?"

"It's what Dr. Ahmed prescribed."

"No, it sure is not! Where did you get that name from? There's a whiskey called Jim Beam, I think, and it certainly can't be taken as a medicine!"

"That's why I came home, because I was supposed to get it in the hospital but they wouldn't give it to me. You're just in denial again." This happened at least a half dozen times in the three days of her pass. Then she lamented over and over and over again about her platelets: *"The Elliston Unit is a psych unit. I'm not supposed to be there. My platelet mobility is the only problem. They're sticking. They're only thirty-eight over forty-four. You don't care if I die."* Each evening the darkened and locked bathroom tyranny continued as before. Each day Kaija spent most of the time lying on the bed upstairs; I could hear her responding

to her voices loudly, angrily, as before. Twice she talked with Taivaan Valtion Isa in Finnish. At least these were happy conversations. The second morning, in contrast, she woke me up, crying, *"I'm crying because I said 'paska'* (shit) *and that's swearing and I shouldn't have said that, I didn't mean to, and now these people are all nattering at me and I just want to sleep but they keep on and on about it."*

Later that day, when I came back from getting groceries, she was again in tears, this time in the kitchen. She looked so woebegone that I almost cried, too.

"Why are you crying, hon?"

"Because they were going to keep you in the store for three months."

That evening after I returned from visiting Kaija's father in the care home (Kaija would not go with me) I once more found her in tears, *"because they weren't going to let you come home from there, ever."*

I took some comfort in knowing that she still loved me and was afraid that I would be taken from her. It was small comfort, however, for her fears and tears were not of this world, but only related to her world of hallucinations and "ad lib," to her psychosis that had already separated us long ago.

The most trying was Kaija's insistence, right from the start, that "I'm not going back to the Elliston Wing." I couldn't count how many times she reiterated this same adamant refrain. And the excuses slid off her tongue like quick silver: *"There's no bed there for me anymore ... They'll keep me there for 243 days ... I can't get pills for my platelets there ... I'm not going back today; I can stay home till tomorrow night ... If I go back they'll keep me for 334 days and I can't get my Wellbutrin in there ... Why do you want me to go back? Is it just that you need a break from me? ... They only have a small cubicle without air conditioning there for me ... Dr. Ahmed just said I don't have to come back ... I don't need to be in any psych wing; there's nothing wrong with my mind ... "*

I can just imagine how much fun it's going to be to get her to go back, I thought.

And sure enough, it was as much a challenge as every other time. I kept talking to her about it, gently, as evening came and the dreaded hour for her return drew near. I was trying to get her used to the idea, and it seemed to be working at first. She slowly showed signs of acquiescence, first by getting out of bed, then, after a while, by dressing and coming downstairs. However, when I came in after surreptitiously loading her stuff into the car, I found her undressed and back in bed! She had even hung her clothes back in the closet instead of on the hook behind the door as she usually did.

And so I started all over. For forty-five minutes I talked first gently, then firmly, and finally Kaija put on her clothes "only so I can go out on the deck for a smoke." I quickly took advantage of that, went out with her, and locked the door behind me, as I had done before. But no amount of talking would persuade her. I finally called Lars and Lillian, and Esther and Walter to drive in to Riverview and try to help persuade her. They were met with a veritable storm of verbal abuse for a full ten minutes, but finally she must have seen the futility of her resistance and without saying a word, got into the car.

As her brother and sister and spouses went to bid her good-bye, she suddenly mellowed and asked them to forgive her. How tender her true heart really was. I couldn't hold back my tears. This was my real wife. This was the real Kaija. This was my sweetheart. Before I backed out of the driveway, she leaned over and asked me to forgive her, too. I did.

Chapter 17: What Next?

Dr. Ahmed was very disappointed to hear how the home pass had gone.

"I don't know what to do," he lamented. "We've tried almost everything there is to try and nothing seems to be working. And we're still treating symptoms, not a specific illness that can be clearly defined."

"I've done some more reading on the Internet," I replied, "and although I know you don't like to categorize, she was diagnosed by Dr. McRae in the beginning as having a psychotic depression. When I checked this out, the CPA listed symptoms such as suicidal thoughts, intellectual impairment, hypochondria, audio or visual hallucination, aggression, frustration, agitation, hopelessness, constipation, and insomnia. Here's the list."

"So what is your point? How many of these symptoms do you think Kaija has?"

"I don't think she has the first three or the last three. That leaves only four out of ten. Well, perhaps there is some intellectual impairment in that she gets confused, as she sometimes says, yet her memory is 100 percent and when she's at her best, her thinking and general knowledge and understanding are just as sharp as ever."

"Well, of course different symptoms apply to different people, and some symptoms overlap and are common to many psychoses."

"I know. It seems to me, though, that she has more of the given symptoms for schizophrenia than for PD. Out of many symptoms listed, she clearly has these ten: hearing internal voices; believing others can invade her mind; paranoia from critical voices; anxiety; fearfulness; withdrawal from social relationships; no insight into her illness, or no distinctions between the real world and the imaginary world; hostility; confusion; and delusions."

"Well, I have seen most of these in Kaija, yet they overlap with many other psychoses. And we don't like to use the term 'schizophrenia' nowadays because of the negative and wrong impressions people have gotten of it from the horror movies such as *Psycho, Silence of the Lambs,* and so on. These always depict the most extreme cases, and people have come to attribute any severely irrational behavior as schizophrenia."

"My only concern is that if Kaija has not been diagnosed correctly, she may not be getting the most effective treatment."

"I don't think you have to worry about that. We're treating a psychosis, and the medications we've tried are used in most cases. I do agree that we don't have a clear diagnosis yet, and maybe we never will have. But I want to do some more testing to at least rule out some possible causes such as vascular dementia or hyperthyroidism or some neurological interference. Now that she's back in the hospital, I plan to do a number of these to try to come to an understanding of what caused the psychosis. If we can find this out, then we can treat a specific illness or disorder."

Dr. Ahmed was certainly more thorough in trying to track down the cause of Kaija's psychosis than the other two psychiatrists had been. He was as good as his word. Over a three-week period Kaija was given various tests. Dr. Ahmed had another EEG run. It was a big word, but I again resorted to the Internet to be reminded that an electroencephalography measured electrical activity in the brain to determine various brain function abnormalities such as epileptic seizures or even brain death. This was followed by a SPEC scan (single photon emission computed tomography), an injection of a radioactive substance, showing which brain tissues used a lot of blood, thus helping determine which bits of the brain were active, or which may be cancerous.

There was more geriatric testing, seeking specifically to what degree Kaija might have vascular dementia, a common ailment that comes with aging. From what I could understand, there were many causes for such dementia, and basically the tests measured the condition of the blood vessels and blood flow to the brain.

Following extensive blood tests (I couldn't count how many blood tests Kaija had had over the past year) there were interviews and consultations with an endocrinologist to measure for hyper- or hypothyroidism. One of them, I couldn't remember which, had a strange name: "Hashimoto's disease." Perhaps because the word sounded like Quasimoto, the name of the hunchback character in Victor Hugo's *The Hunchback of Notre Dame*, it had a strong negative connotation for me and I hoped Kaija did not have such a disease. The tests showed borderline hypothyroidism, not serious enough to warrant treatment.

The report from Kaija's examination by a neuropsychologist gave me a much-needed chuckle. How long ago had it been since I had had such a good laugh? I wondered. The report at first made me feel good. Here was a woman who recognized Kaija's "genius," as I liked to call it. It opened with, "Thank you for referring this fascinating woman to me for consultation … She is a very high-functioning woman … who had no mental health problems until recently." Then, near the end of the report was the really hilarious statement, "Kaija is a very heavy alcohol user and may have had withdrawal symptoms when she was first admitted. Apparently, she likes Jack Daniels."

I hadn't laughed so hard since I read Frank McCourt's novels, *Angela's Ashes* and *'Tis*. My dear Kaija had never drank alcohol, let alone been an alcoholic! It sure showed how very real her hallucinations were, how convincing she could be when talking about them, and how the wall separating reality from fantasy had completely dissolved. She had obviously related her Jim Beam (or Jim Bream, as she usually called it) obsession to the neuropsychologist and had taken her in completely. On top of that, I guffawed over the Jack Daniels statement; Kaija had never spoken that brand name, and likely would not even know what it was.

The upshot of all the testing was—nothing! Still no obvious causes of the psychosis. Still nothing to treat but the symptoms. Still no insights into what treatments or medications would be most effective. It was frustrating, not only to me but to Dr. Ahmed as well.

"At least she's doing better now in the hospital, so maybe the combination of Zyprexa and Zydis is beginning to have a positive effect. I'll be gone on vacation for three weeks, and I think it's best that we keep Kaija on the same meds and dosage as she's been on since coming in here."

Then Dr. Ahmed dropped the bombshell.

"In any case, we have to start considering some other option for Kaija other than going from hospital to home and home to hospital. Obviously this is not working, yet we can't keep her in the hospital indefinitely. There's always a shortage of beds, and besides, the hospital setting with all its commotion and interruptions is not the best place for her to be. But home isn't, either, as we have seen. I think it's time you start looking for other options, for some kind of long-term care facility. We should aim for mid-August. That's not a firm date, but it's six weeks from the date of her re-entry. The psychiatric ward is not a long-term facility; we generally try for a six- to eight-week turnaround. The aim is to stabilize patients within those six weeks and then move them back into their former environment or into a suitable long-term facility."

My heart sank. I hadn't expected this. I thought that Kaija would be kept in the hospital until she improved enough to come home again. I realized that this had not worked out well in the past, but I was counting on the new meds to have a better effect than the earlier ones. Perhaps I was relying on medications to be the magic that would lead Kaija to an acceptable level of recovery in order to remain at home. But what else was there? I had considered homeopathy.

"What do you think of homeopathic treatment?" I asked Dr. Ahmed.

"Well, no one has all the answers ... but if you want to try it, just let me know what she will be taking so that there won't be any conflict of medications."

But I, myself, had no faith in homeopathy. I knew a number of relatives and friends that were getting very expensive homeopathic treatments for all kinds of things. The treatments were so complex, the products so numerous, that I knew that I would never be able to keep Kaija on such a program, let alone convince her to even see a homeopath. Furthermore, I could not see that my friends' treatments had ever had more than a temporary effect, much as a placebo often has.

Then there were all the health food miracle products in which I had no faith at all. The more I checked into them, the more convinced I was that many of them were just money-making schemes. Kaija and I had at one time or another tried a few of them, but they had all been bogus and had not helped one bit. Vitamins were not much better, in spite of the claims that were made for them. Yes, perhaps some like vitamin D and vitamin C were helpful in specific situations, but for all the years that I had taken multivitamins, for example, I could not recall a single instance when I felt that they were improving my health one bit.

So, where did all that leave me? It seemed to me that Dr. Ahmed was looking now at something nonmedical as a way to alleviate Kaija's psychosis, something in addition to the medications. A quiet place. A place away from her too-familiar home atmosphere. A place where she could be treated passively, that would offer her some peace from daily pressures and concerns. A place away from the noisy psychiatric ward. A place away from me.

Chapter 18: Psychotic Systems and People

My heart was heavy. The thought of placing Kaija in some sort of long-term care facility seemed like such a final act. To do so, it seemed to me, was to write her off, to get rid of her, because she would never be the same again. To get rid of her because she was cluttering up my life. To get rid of her because I was not strong enough, or resilient enough, to adjust to the changes in our lives and to cope with the unknowns of the immediate future—the "betwixt and between" state that Grace, in Vanderhaeghe's *The Englishman's Boy,* talks about.

I shouldn't have even brought her back here, I thought. I should have bitten the bullet and learned to cope with Kaija in one way or another. Am I really such a crappy husband that I can't even take care of my own wife? Why am I even on Lamotrigine if it doesn't help me enough to cope emotionally? I shouldn't even need such a crutch. I'm healthy. I'm four years younger than Kaija; it's my place to look after her. Am I just another immoral degenerate of the "me generation"? Shouldn't I just bring her back home?

I felt as though the blood had just drained out of me. My legs felt like rubber. My heart pounded. I felt that I was going to faint.

Dr. Ahmed must have read my mind, but my thoughts were likely imprinted on my features and evident in my psychosomatic reaction.

"You shouldn't kick yourself over a decision like this. It's a natural part of the healing process whenever a patient does not respond immediately to treatment. We, and you, have certainly tried our best, over more than a year already, to counter her illness at least enough so that she could remain at home. So far, we've failed to do so. Now we must try something different. You've done all you can. You can see that in spite of your best intentions, in spite of your deep love for your wife (which I've noticed, by the way), you are unable to help her now in her present condition. You need to move on now, to take another step on the journey to recovery and do what is best for Kaija, and also for you."

"Don't try to shift the focus onto me! I'll come through this one way or another. I'm my mother's son and I don't give up that easily. It's just that this seems like such a callous thing to do. And I'd sooner live with an ill Kaija than no Kaija at all."

"Did I say this would be forever?"

"No, I guess you didn't, but it seems to me that it will be."

"Nonsense. I still think we can help Kaija recover, not 100 percent but a long way toward it. I have faith that over a few more weeks the Zyprexa, especially, will begin to have an effect. I'd say we should give it another four or five months, but that we augment its effectiveness by having her in an environment that is more conducive to healing. I think you can see the benefit of that. And I think you're strong enough to live apart from her for that long. It doesn't mean you can't visit her, though I don't think you should do so right away. She'll need time to settle in and begin to accept her new home. If you go there right away, she'll just be upset when you don't take her home."

I took a deep breath. "OK. But where am I to start? What kinds of facilities are there? And where?"

"You need to speak to one of the social workers about that. But I'd recommend a personal care home over a mental health care home. The latter would not be a good environment for Kaija; most of the clients in such homes are in worse condition than she is. But don't you worry about that yet; I'll arrange for you to meet with a social worker tomorrow. Can you stay in the city?"

"Of course. I'm not working, and I'm here to do whatever I can to help Kaija."

Thus began my latest nightmare—seeking somewhere to place Kaija. Just to think of it made it seem as though I was trying to find a home for a pet dog that I could no longer keep. I met the next day with Rachel, a social worker. She was young, with a pleasant and welcoming smile and a soft, yet direct look in her eyes. She made me feel at ease immediately. We had a long talk about Kaija's and my situation. Rachel was understanding, empathetic, helpful. It soon became evident that I would likely have to look for some kind of a care home in the city, for in our own Prairie West Health District there were only care homes for the elderly. Still, Rachel suggested that I talk to the Prairie West administrators to see if they provided rooms for special situations such as intermediate-term respite. She informed me that there were many such government-approved and supported facilities in the city, too, and that this may be a better option as Kaija would be closer to follow-up care with her psychiatrist and her assigned social worker.

Private personal care homes were another option. Rachel gave me a thick booklet listing all the ones in the city and surrounding towns. It also listed private mental care homes, and Rachel explained the difference between the two. Kaija may be eligible for one or the other, depending on the level of both her physical and mental needs.

As the talk progressed, I discovered I now had three different hoops I would have to jump through. The first was that the onus was on me to find a suitable, and available, home for Kaija. As I paged through the listings in the booklet Rachel had given me, I was overwhelmed by the number of them and by the variations in size, amenities, and restrictions that each listed. Where was I to start? What was the procedure? Would contact be first made by the social worker, or was I to contact each one directly? Could I just drive up and ask to see the facility and talk to the owner/operator? Or did I have to make an appointment? Did I have to have a referral from a nurse, doctor, or administrator of the Elliston Wing? Did I need approval from the psychiatrist for my choice? I felt like a beached fish floundering in a catch pool, struggling to survive until the next wave, hopefully, would return me to my familiar and safe environment.

The second hoop, before I could even consider finding a place, was to have Kaija "evaluated, to determine what level she's at and to find out what her needs are, what kinds of care she will require." That meant, first of all, that a social worker would interview Kaija to get an understanding of her mental condition, and then begin to check listings of appropriate homes. She would then give this narrowed-down list to me for follow-up. Secondly, Kaija would be interviewed and evaluated by an occupational therapist to determine what she was capable of doing on her own, and what kind of training might be necessary to help her become more self-sufficient over time. Finally, she would have to have a Daily Living Support Assessment to determine what level of care was required, which would then be used to place her in the proper kind of facility.

The result of the first interview was that if a retirement home was not feasible, Kaija would definitely have to be placed in a private mental health care home (just the opposite of what Dr. Ahmed had thought!), which was different, the interviewer explained, from a private personal care home. The former took in only patients with mental health problems, whereas the latter did not accept anyone with mental health issues but only those that needed help because of physical infirmities. This narrowed down the list of possible placements considerably, but as it turned out, at present there were no openings in any of the mental care home facilities. The social worker would let me know when any openings came available.

"Does that mean that I have to accept the first one

that comes open, since the staff at the Elliston Wing want her out within two weeks?" I asked.

"No, certainly not. The mid-August date they gave you at City Hospital is not that firm; it's a target date, but they can force you neither to take Kaija back home if she has not improved considerably nor to place her in any other unsuitable environment."

"So she can stay in the Elliston Wing until I can find her a suitable place?"

"Yes, it's kind of a conditional thing, the conditions being the state of her mental health week by week, the availability of beds, and the fact that you are actively searching for a home and are in agreement that this is the best option for Kaija at this time."

"So I gather that you will let me know when there are any openings in private mental health care homes so that I don't have to try and track this by myself? And that I don't necessarily have to accept the first one that becomes available?"

"That's right. I'm here to help you with that task and those decisions."

The occupational therapy assessment seemed like a Mickey Mouse exercise to me. It measured "visuo-spatial perception and executive functioning." Kaija made it clear that the executive clock-drawing task, the first one on the test, was childish, and of course she scored fifteen out of fifteen on it.

The second part, the Executive Interview, revealed nothing new but merely reaffirmed what the medical professional and I had known for a long time: "Kaija showed impairment of executive functioning … difficulty being spontaneous, disinhibition, and perseveration

... She scored 13/50, which places her in the 'mild impairment' category."

The third evaluation, the Daily Living Support Assessment overlapped the OT one in many of the questions that were put to Kaija. However, it was more comprehensive, and its objective was to determine an official level of care on a rating scale from one to five, with one indicating minimal care and five indicating complete care. This rating would determine what kind of facility would accept Kaija.

The test had many, many subcategories, but basically measured performance under four major categories: dependence, behavior, health, and independent living. Kaija scored very low on independent living skills—no surprise. Overall she was rated a level IV. I was taken aback; I didn't think Kaija was that bad. I mentioned this to Ethan, the examiner. He was a rather brusque, no nonsense sort of guy, and his response was that he had done hundreds of these tests and the results were pretty accurate. It seemed to me that Kaija was just a piece of paper to him, yet I understood that he did not know her as I did, and that from his perspective and the results of the test, she really was a level IV. But it hurt me to think so. He said he would pass this information on to Rachel, the social worker, so that she could focus on homes that accepted level-IV patients.

The third, and surely the most frustrating, of the three hoops (after I had found out the costs of the various homes) was to find out if there were any kinds of government subsidies to help meet such costs. I quickly learned that care homes for the elderly ran from eleven hundred to thirteen hundred dollars per month, but varied somewhat depending on the patient's income. If income was derived from only Old Age Pension and CPP, then the cost might be as much as a hundred dollars less. Private care homes, both personal and mental, cost $1401 per month. The one dollar above fourteen hundred dollars made me laugh. Were they trying to legitimize the exorbitant cost by making it seem as if the actual costs were calculated to the dollar? I wondered what the profit margin was—30 percent ... 50 percent ... more? The only cost I could see was the food, and minimal amounts for laundry and bath soap; all notions, clothing, or any special needs were the patient's responsibility. Of course, one had to factor in some utility costs, but these could not be much since the homes were also the permanent dwellings of the caregivers. That would make a tidy sum, I thought. Even in a home with only five patients, which was common, the gross income would be over seven thousand dollars a month. Not bad for someone with only minimal training.

Fourteen hundred dollars was a big bite for me now that I wasn't working steadily. Employment insurance paid only 60 percent of my salary, and even that would come to an end soon. I didn't regret that I had stayed home to look after Kaija, but if I had to pay that amount for a longer time, I'd have to try to find another teaching job—and they were scarcer than robins in winter. I hoped I wouldn't have to draw out our RRSPs at this age.

The social workers (two of them) and the Prairie West Mental Health nurse had all told me that yes, there were programs to subsidize the costs if one was in need of such. But when I tried to get specific information I ran into a bureaucratic jungle. I phoned what seemed the most likely government department to handle such issues, but was shunted to another ... then to another ... and another. Altogether I made thirteen calls. The last was to a Central Intake department through which "all applications for aid are channeled." They began by doing an initial interview over the phone. What a joke that turned out to be! After answering only a half dozen questions, it became clear that this was the final dead end. Basically, it was an application for social assistance under any circumstances, and to qualify one could be earning no more than fifteen hundred dollars a month—in other words, one had to be destitute. Well, though I was far from well off, I was not that poor, so I cut the interview short.

A brain wave hit me after that—a shortsighted one, I realized later, for it meant Kaija would be at home, and they had agreed that this was not a good plan at all right now. But I momentarily forgot that in my focus on funding Kaija's care. I made one more call—to the provincial Ministry of Health.

"Look," I explained to the minister himself, "I've phoned every social agency in the province to try and get financial help to cover the cost of having my wife in a private care home. After being given the runaround for three days, I appeal to you. Since it costs the government about two hundred dollars a day to keep a patient in a hospital ..."

"You mean more like six hundred to eight hundred dollars a day ..."

"Well, that makes my point even stronger. Wouldn't it make sense for you to pay me just fifty or a hundred dollars a day to stay home and look after my wife.

Think of the savings for Sask Health and the people of Saskatchewan if this were the case. I'm likely only one of thousands in this situation …"

"But that's not the way we look at it. The government's position is that health care is the family's responsibility first, and we don't pay for that. We come in only after family options and efforts have been exhausted."

There was no use in pursuing it any further. I could smell a bureaucratic rat as easily as the next person. It was clear from the minister's overconfident, know-it-all tone of voice that he wouldn't give a moment's thought to the idea. But where was the logic in the minister's position? Yes, I agreed family responsibility was first, and I had been giving that—as much of myself as I possibly could—for the past fifteen months. Now it was no longer possible; nevertheless, I was suggesting a way that I could continue to do so, at huge savings to the government. It would be simple to devise and administer a plan with checks and balances to avoid abuse of the plan.

There seemed to be an affinity between government and psychosis—neither had any understanding of logic.

So, perhaps it had been a subconscious act of desperation for me to consider having Kaija at home again since the doctor would not even allow it. That fact had been suppressed in my deep-down desire to have her at home. That's how life itself tended to be; the positive moments were at the fore more often than the negative ones, at least for me. I believed in Wordsworth's "moments recollected in tranquility" that brought back the past so vividly that it was like reliving a particular, happy moment all over again. My life with Kaija had been such that the difficult moments seemed few in comparison to the happiness we had shared. My love for her had not diminished one whit because of this psychosis; if anything, it had been renewed and strengthened by my need to protect and care for her. But would there ever be true happiness in our lives again?

It was with a heavy heart that I set up an appointment with Prairie West Health to see what care facilities existed in our own district. I had already found out that there were only two private personal care homes, and both accepted elderly patients of sound mind only

My meeting with Cheryl Harvey, head of Prairie West District Health Services, unnerved me for two reasons. The first was that she didn't seem to want to even consider Kaija's case. She knew the situation well, since she had been in charge of the home care nurses that had given Kaija her meds when she was at home last spring.

"The care homes in our district are all homes for the elderly. Kaija doesn't fit that demographic …"

"She's almost reached retirement age," I blurted out. "You can't dismiss her just like that. I know one of the patients in the home here very well; she's only sixty-two and she's been here for two years already. I know that some of her problems are mental, too."

"I can't discuss individual cases here …"

"I know that, and I didn't use any names, but I just made the reference to make the point that Kaija …"

"Each case is different. We evaluate each one on its own merits, so comparisons don't even enter the picture. There's a long list of criteria that we examine …"

"OK, so why do you assume that Kaija would not qualify?"

"I know Kaija's situation very well. She's too mentally

unstable, and we don't take patients with obvious psychoses; the only ones with mental problems that we accept are the elderly, those with dementia, Alzheimer's, and so on."

"But Kaija, according to Dr. Ahmed, is not impaired enough to go into a mental health care home, so that's why I thought this might be an option …"

"Well, you know, a leopard can't change its spots …"

Of all the ignorant statements, I thought, that is the most ignorant I've ever heard. I was seething. This woman obviously did not even understand that recovery from psychoses was possible … Ah, what was the use even thinking about it. I was too angry to even think straight.

The second thing that unnerved me was a statement by Cheryl Harvey's assistant: "I can give you one bit of information that will answer your question when you phoned earlier asking about costs and whether there is any financial assistance. There isn't, really, but there is one way you can get some help."

"What's that?"

"You can apply for a legal separation."

"Are you kidding? I have no intention of separating just because …"

"Hold on. This doesn't mean that you actually separate for good. It's specifically for "involuntary separation," situations where because of health or other reasons beyond their control a couple is forced to live apart. It's simply a financial, on-paper arrangement that allows you to receive a Guaranteed Income Supplement paid to each of you as a single person. Right now, if you receive a GIS, it's based on your marital status and your total income as a couple."

"Well, Kaija already started receiving a small Guaranteed Income Supplement last year, but I'm not of retirement age yet, so I don't understand where the benefit lies."

"What will happen is that Kaija's GIS will likely double or triple. Since she is not earning any money besides her Old Age Pension and CPP, her income is very low. And since yours was high when you were teaching, her GIS was very low or nil because it was based on both of your earnings together. If you take your earnings out of the equation, then Kaija will qualify for much more, since the GIS is a supplement to the Old Age Pension and the amount received is based on annual earnings. In most cases where we've seen this happen, the amount of increase is usually enough to cover the costs of residency in a care home facility."

"I sure don't like the sound of that at all. Legal separation makes it sound as though it's a forever thing …"

"No, it's not. Remember, it's just a legal paper allowing you to claim separate incomes, nothing more that that. You'll still be married. That does not change. Then, if you're able to live together again after a while, whether it's a few months or a few years, you simply notify the government and they change the supplement based, again, on your combined incomes."

"Well, they could sure call it something else; the connotation is terrible. If I told any of my family that we were legally separated, they'd have a fit."

"You don't even have to tell anybody about it. It's as

private and personal as your income taxes. It is a monetary arrangement, not a moral issue. Here, I'll give you the forms, you can read over the details and instructions, and then it's entirely up to you whether you apply or not. No one, not even the Health Care officials, have to know anything about it."

"OK, I'll look it over and give it some thought. And thanks! It's the only specific information and help I've received yet in my quest for financial aid programs. Not even the minister of health told me about this one."

"I wish you well in your search for a home for Kaija. And maybe it will only be for a short time."

"Yeah. But I feel somewhat like a boll weevil nevertheless."

Psychotic systems, I thought, yet maybe no more paranoid or psychotic than I am with my jump-the-gun reaction to this legal separation business. One thing I knew for sure: I would be married to Kaija "till death do us part," as I had promised.

Chapter 19: Still Roller Coasting

"I won't cry, you'll see. Just take me home from here, even if it's only for a three-day pass."

Such a plaintive cry! It tore at my heart. I wanted to gather Kaija in my arms and just walk out the door of the Elliston Wing with her. How could I say no to her? Yet I had to. I didn't know if Dr. Ahmed had completed all the testing he wanted to do, and of course I could not take her home without a pass from him.

Leaving this time was one of the worst torture sessions I had gone through yet. But my tortured feelings were likely mild compared to those of Kaija. She cried and cried, and begged and begged me to take her home. But it couldn't be, not now. As the parting moment came, we held one another so hard. Through our mingled tears we blessed one another.

"You won't commit suicide, will you?" Kaija read my desperation correctly. She was afraid, after seeing me so in despair. But I assured her I would not even think of it, and I walked out into the night.

When I visited the next day, Dr. Ahmed had a surprise for me.

"I will be away for three weeks starting tomorrow. Dr. Balamani will look after Kaija while I'm away. We won't be doing any more testing, and Kaija can stay on the same meds. We need to give the Zyprexa much more time. It seems to me that at times it is already having some positive effect. So I want you to try again. Take Kaija home on a three-day pass, and then let Dr. Balamani know how it goes."

And so, as July gave way to August, with much trepidation I took Kaija home on a pass. I didn't think the four weeks in the Elliston Wing had done much good, but the nurses had told me that the good moments were outweighing the bad.

And they were, even at home. Oh, not all was peaches and cream, but it was obvious that Kaija was much better than she had been before her admission. I kept detailed notes in my journal so that I could give an accurate picture to Dr. Balamani.

Thursday
Kaija was extremely happy to be coming home. She was so with it on the drive home, commenting on the colors of the trees and the crops, on the meadowlarks' warble from atop the fence posts, and many other things. She was as delighted as a little child at first discovery of nature's marvels ... Did not go to lie down right away as usual ... Reminisced about her Toronto days ... Read the newspaper ... Went for a short walk together ... Sat on the deck, smoking and chatting ... Only one *"Be quiet"* when getting ready for bed, but had the light off as usual ...

Friday
Fairly good day ... Visited well with Esther and Walter over AM coffee ... Visited with her dad in the retirement home for thirty-five minutes ... Enjoyed meals, thanking me with a kiss each time ... Helped clear up after ... Peaceful and smiley all PM, though she rested upstairs most of the time ... A few laments about Lars poking her ...

Saturday
Good day! Happy, emotionally alive, eyes bright, real smiles ... Read a lot of the newspaper ... Went willingly to Esther and Walter's for supper and evening visit; very alive and normal there, even laughing a lot ... Had stomach cramps after supper, so lay down and cried 'cause *"Lars is poking my stomach ..."*

Sunday
Said in PM that *"we're supposed to go to Esther's for meatball supper."* Actually not, but she phoned and of course Esther said, "Sure, come on over." Animated there ... Went to evening church and visited with lots of people, though conversations were short ...

Monday
Another good day, though mostly rested ... Visited with Rebecca, our niece, and enjoyed looking at her maritime pics ... Helped me make Nanking cherry jelly ... Went for an ice cream. Really enjoyed it ...

Overall, it was a good weekend. As she had promised, Kaija did not cry. I had not seen her in such good form for ages and ages. I faxed my notes to Dr. Balamani so that he would have them to look over before we met on Tuesday.

Whatever unspoken dreams and hopes I had during the past four days, however, vanished when it came time to take Kaija back.

"I'm not going back," she shouted, and hit me twice on the top of my head with her fist. "I'm not going. You can't make me!"

For the next half hour this scene, these words, were repeated over and over. Kaija would not give in. I tried every trick in my repertoire, but nothing had even the slightest effect. In desperation I did what I had to do before, so against my will: I called for an ambulance.

Kaija's reaction to the ambulance personnel was the same—shouts of "I won't go" over and over as she lay huddled under the quilt on our bed. It was the same nightmare all over again. Finally, I called 911 and had them send over two police officers. Once again, I managed to trick Kaija by saying, "OK, lets go out for a smoke," and as before, I then locked the door behind us.

Kaija greeted the police with the same shouts, but now she added excuse after excuse, *"I don't need to go back. They released me right after I was admitted ... I would have been home long ago but Charles would not come and get me ... The only thing wrong with me is that my platelets are low and they can't fix them there. It's a psych hospital and there's nothing wrong with my mind ... They don't have a bed for me ..."*

There were numerous other excuses, but I could not remember them all. The police kept talking gently but firmly. "You'll have to go, one way or another. We don't like to force you, but it's not our call. The doctor has not released you to stay at home indefinitely, and so legally you must return. You don't see it this way, but we are here to do what is best for you ... So, shall we go now?"

Finally, Kaija relented by saying, "I can't go in these clothes."

"I'll get your jeans and a T-shirt. You can change in the bathroom downstairs," I said.

I brought the clothes downstairs and let Kaija into the house, but not before I asked one of the policemen to guard the entry to the living room so that she could not head upstairs. As she came back out onto the deck, one of the policemen asked, "Would you rather go with Charles than with us?"

"Yes, I'd rather go with Charles," Kaija answered meekly. She got into the car. As the police and ambulance pulled away, Kaija asked me to forgive her for being so angry. I did, of course, and as we headed for the city the popular gospel song, "Will the Circle Be Unbroken," went round and round in my head, driving me half crazy.

* * *

Another appeal hearing was held the next morning to determine if Kaija had to stay in the hospital, and if so, to get the authorization to keep her against her will. I was astounded at Dr. Balamani's report.

"In my opinion, Kaija need not stay in the hospital. We will not be doing any more testing right now or changing any of her medications. I feel she will respond better to the medications in her home environment than here in a hospital setting. Charles' report, which he sent me yesterday, says that Kaija was exceptionally good over the past four days at home …"

"That's true, but what I have not had time to tell you is how difficult it was for me to get her to return when the pass was over. I had to call the ambulance and the police to get her to comply. So yes, she was much better, but the episode at the end makes me leery about having her at home again so soon. Are you sure it's the right thing to do?"

"I do, in spite of the difficulty of getting her to come back. That's a natural reaction and I don't see it as a strong psychotic response to the situation. Of course she would rather be at home than in here ..."

"I'll be good," Kaija interjected. "I won't get angry as long as I don't need to come back into this place."

"I suppose you're right, Doctor, and I would like her to be at home, too, but the ferocity of her refusal to return dismayed and scared me. I don't know if I can handle it if she should behave in this way again."

I hated having to talk about Kaija in this way while she sat there listening to the whole discussion. It was almost as though she was not even present, and I found this not only disconcerting but rude. But Kaija was so impassive; she offered so little in her defense that I wondered if she really was able to follow the conversation. Other than her one comment about being good, she remained detached and aloof and appeared to not pay any attention to the discussion of her condition. As had happened a million times, I just could not comprehend her behavior. I would have expected her to give an animated, emotional appeal for release but she just sat there, just as inaccessible now, in this state, as when she was over the edge in a full-blown psychotic episode. Such emotional unresponsiveness (lack of affect was what the psychiatrists called it) was another of the classic symptoms of schizophrenia, so I guess I shouldn't have been surprised.

"But until the time to return she was very good. I think that if she stays on these same medications, she will continue to improve. If my hypothesis is correct, do you think you could manage it?"

"Yes, I guess so. I don't want to make it sound like I'm trying to get rid of her by having her stay in the hospital. I'm confused, though, because Dr. Ahmed advised me to begin looking for a care home for her."

"Well, at this stage, we don't even know if it's definitely a psychosis we're treating. I think there might also be vascular degeneration, and in that case, there is little we could do in the hospital."

That also astounded me. Vascular degeneration, Dr. Lewis had explained to me long ago, led to dementia and usually did not occur at this age. I had long ago ruled it out. It did not at all fit into Kaija's behavior pattern, especially since she could be so lucid quite often. It irked me that a doctor who had little knowledge of Kaija's situation could just come up with his own diagnoses based on the little he had seen her. I doubted that Dr. Balamani had even had time to read through her file.

I would have argued and tried to refute Dr. Balamani's theories, but I felt that this was not the time or place to do it. I'd speak to him after the hearing. I was pretty sure the decision would follow the pattern of all of the earlier ones and the committee would deny Kaija a release from hospital care.

Once more, I was taken aback. Only a half hour later Dr. Balamani came to Kaija's room, smiling. "You've won your appeal! You can go home today. This is not just a short pass. We're releasing you to remain at home indefinitely."

I could not even be happy about the decision. I had gone through so many tough experiences with Kaija, and since the latest and one of the hardest had been just yesterday, I was not at all confident that such behavioral eruptions wouldn't occur again. The ambulance/police scenarios drove me crazy. As "crazy" as Kaija? I wondered. In a different way, yes. They made me so emotionally overwrought, frustrated, angry ... and guilty at having to treat my wife this way. I did not want a repeat performance. Although I hated to admit it, I had learned by experience that it was easier to live apart than amidst such turmoil. I was not at all confident that four days of good behavior were indicative of the next few weeks' behavior. But then again, if the meds were starting to work ...

"Let's go pack your stuff, hon. You're outta here and coming home. Are you glad?"

"Of course I'm glad!" Big smile. Eyes aglow. Voice animated. Step light and bouncy. This was my real wife, the one I had seen so little of these past fifteen months. I shook my head. I could not understand. How could there be such contrasts? She was forever surprising me with her changing behavior pattern. Which Kaija was I really taking home—the old or the new? The ill or the healthy? Or both?

Chapter 20: Will It Ever End?

We had been home barely ten minutes. *"Will you get me that Jules Bream now?"*

It was to be a refrain repeated daily, and sometimes Kaija nearly drove me crazy with her insistence on having it.

"No. Don't get into that again or you'll be back in the hospital toute de suite." I hated myself for threatening her this way, and I had read that this was not an acceptable way to relate to someone with schizophrenia, but my exasperation knew no bounds. Same old, same old! Would she harass me with this same request every day? Would I have to face her anger and tears every day? Where was that good behavior now? Why had it departed, and so soon? How was I to comprehend such radically changing behavior? How was I supposed to deal with it? After all this time, I felt just as ignorant, just as helpless, as ever.

"There are many bottles of it in the big black suitcase under the stairs," Kaija confidently asserted one time. *"But it's too heavy for me so you'll have to get it for me."*

As the days wore on she became more and more

insistent, more and more angry with me, more and more creative in her appeals.

"Are you going to get me that Jim Bream now? It's the only medicine that will help my platelets. You are so stupid ... For nine months I've been sick, nine months I've gone without it because of you, nine months you've been in denial ... You're so cold-hearted. You just want me to die ... We have to go to Esther's so she can start me on that Jim Beam. Jon Kangas said all the Finns drink alcohol for their platelets. He's a doctor, so he should know ... Esther is at the Liquor Board store getting it now ... It's in the car trunk. Go and get it right now ... I need four ounces in the morning, four at two o'clock, then another four at bedtime ... Elina took it for six months and she got better ... The adult dose is four ounces with two ounces of orange juice at eight, ten, twelve, two, four, and six, with a chaser at bedtime ... We're booked into the Hilton, room 106. They gave us a good rate, just 560 dollars for a week. You can start me on Jack Beam there ... "

It was a case of history repeating itself for two weeks. Many days Kaija packed her clothes into plastic bags (I kept the suitcases locked in the car trunk) to *"go to Esther's so I can start on Jack Bream,"* or *"go to the Hilton"* or *"go to the new house."*

Her smoking obsession became more and more dominant. *"Dr. Naipaul said I have to have a smoke at eight fifteen, nine fifteen, and ten fifteen so I get enough tar into my system to keep my heart from fibrillating ... I'm supposed to smoke thirteen cigarettes a day ... "*

Almost every day she was in tears because *"Lars is poking me."* Every day, many times a day, I would hear her vehemently saying *"Shut up!"* Every evening the bathroom ritual repeated itself: lockdown, lights off, and angry conversations inside. Every day she shouted at me many times for not doing as she bid.

What worried me the most was that more and more often Kaija would become physically abusive. Her anger and frustration spilled over into overt action. It struck me that she had never reacted in a physical way to others. In fact, it's very rare that people with such illnesses do. I was just too familiar to her, I guess, and in her home atmosphere she felt she could give her emotions free reign. Sometimes she would bop me on the head with her fist; at other times, she slugged me, feebly, on the shoulder. Even in the throes of such angry, emotional explosions, I often had to resist the impulse to chuckle. It was just such an absurd contrast in strength, and my poor Kaija's physical efforts were so futile.

As time went on, though, the physical attacks became both more numerous and more violent. She would berate me about being *"stupid"* and *"in denial"* and *"wanting me to die"* and often punch me on the shoulder. Once when she was extremely wrought up, she pinched me on the arm with all her might, and twisted to make it hurt even more. Perhaps it would have, but since I was wearing a thick sweater her efforts remained futile. Her sixth sense must have kicked in and warned her that such violence was not kosher, for she quickly said, *"I was just joking around."*

Kaija knew that violent behavior was not acceptable, for when I would grab her wrists and just hold them, she would never fight back. Usually she would go upstairs, weeping pitifully, but half an hour or an hour later she would come back down, in tears of contrition now, and ask me to forgive her. These moments wrenched my heart far more than the moments of physical abuse. The latter emanated not from my wife, but from the other person that she had become. The tears of contrition, however, were from Kaija's heart, genuine displays of her love for me. I could only fold her in my arms and as silent tears coursed down my face, forgive her. If only this real Kaija would remain! If only … if only …

The home stay ended abruptly, just fifteen days after it had begun. Kaija would not go to her appointment with Dr. Ahmed, so of course there was a Mexican standoff as always. But I had learned to be wily, and I devised a ruse to get her there.

"Our room at the Hilton, that you were talking about earlier, is reserved for tonight. I just checked. So let's head for the city and book in for tonight, but stop by Ahmed's office first to get your prescriptions renewed. You're almost out of pills, and if we're going to stay at the Hilton for a week, you'll need them."

"OK," Kaija replied, all smiles. "I've already got everything packed. My pillow is in this bag, and I even put the daily paper into the overnight bag for you." I didn't bother to remind her that most of the stuff had been packed for many days already.

The appointment at the hospital went as I anticipated. I had faxed my notes regarding Kaija's daily progress the day before to Dr. Ahmed. I felt like a tattletale doing so. I hated to sound so negative. I had tried to keep my notes as factual as possible, blocking out my own emotions; nevertheless, as I read them over, the few positive behaviors were lost in the myriad negative ones.

"I understand your time at home did not go well," Dr. Ahmed said, looking over the notes. "What do you have to say to that?"

"I would have been fine but Charles refused to get me Jim Bream for my platelets. He said you hadn't prescribed it."

"That's true, I didn't. Don't you remember that I told you that is an alcohol, and not a medication? You're already on medication for your platelets ..."

"I am not. You're no better than Charles. You don't care how I feel! I could die and you'd all feel happy."

"Well, I can't give you Jim Beam, but we do have to change your medications, I can see that. And to do that we need to admit you to the hospital so that we can monitor your reaction ..."

"I'm not staying! You can't keep me here! You think I'm crazy and I'm not. I'll never come here again!"

I had to struggle to hold her and keep her from leaving the hospital. I knew now, for sure, that Dr. Ahmed would not let her return home. Her anger, her accusations, her actions had all betrayed her and reinforced what I had written in my notes. Nevertheless, I was jolted by what Dr. Ahmed said next.

"You have to come back into the hospital, but I can admit you only on one condition—that you be transferred to a long-term care home as soon as you are more settled down and not so angry. We can't have you going from hospital to home to hospital and home again like we've been doing. You can't keep driving your poor husband crazy every time you go home, and I can't keep finding you a bed every time on short notice. Going from one place to the other just exacerbates your illness. You need more routine and a more constant, neutral, and peaceful atmosphere. I'm going to ask your husband to start looking for a place right away."

Chapter 21: Kiss of Death

I was completely disheartened by Dr. Ahmed's pronouncement, even though the doctor had discussed this possibility with me earlier. Kaija, by contrast, was affronted and inflamed. That she would not be allowed to return home unhinged her.

"I won't stay here! I will not be admitted! I hate this hospital, and you, too. You just want to put me somewhere to die. You don't care if I ever get better. You've never given me anything for my platelets yet. Anyway, I'm going home right now and you can't stop me. I'd rather die at home than in some place where I'll likely be locked up."

With that, she bolted toward the door. A bulky male nurse was there to stop her. Twice the nurse had to physically restrain Kaija while I went to the car to get her clothes and notions.

As she was led into her room, Kaija's fight left her. She sat on the edge of the bed, limp, dejected, silently weeping, and utterly forlorn. Two broken hearts about to be separated, I thought, perhaps forever. We wept in each other's arms for long, long moments. There was nothing to say. Finally, I took her face in my hands. We looked deep into one another's eyes, and then I kissed her goodbye. I left without looking back.

I returned to Riverview, and the next day began to take the steps that were so against my will. I met with Cheryl Harvey and Sandy McPhee, the Prairie West Health District administrators that morning. They made the necessary phone calls to government officials to get the information and forms for the legal separation. Again they emphasized that this was an "economic separation" only and would not affect our marriage in any way. It was merely a way, the only way, to get some financial aid to help cover the costs of the care home. Kaija's Guaranteed Income Supplement, added to her Old Age Pension, would more than double, and together would cover 75 percent of the care home fee. I felt so crass about the whole affair, yet because I was not working but drawing employment insurance, I needed the extra funds. Financial matters had never concerned me and I had always hated them. I had never let my life be governed by finances, but rather I trusted in the will of God to guide my choices and decisions. But now I felt like a traitor, cold, unfeeling, dead inside. It seemed that I was now letting worry over money dominate in my life. Where did that leave understanding, compassion, love?

I next focused on finding a care home for Kaija.

"Look for a personal care home," Dr. Ahmed had said. "It would not be good for her to be in a mental care home in her state; she's too aware."

I was puzzled by that, for Kaija still had no insight into her illness, and was completely unaware of her seamless shifts from reality to fantasy. And the social worker's tests had definitely rated her a candidate for a mental care home. But it uplifted me a bit, for it seemed that Dr. Ahmed thought that her mental condition was not serious enough to warrant mental care, specifically. Then again, what did I know about the kinds of patients in these homes? Perhaps their states of illness were much more severe than Kaija's, probably like some of those I had seen in the Elliston Wing. No doubt many of them were released into mental care homes to receive adequate, trained, even professional help for their mental illnesses.

I called Glenda McKenzie for some guidance. She apologized for the severe lack of facilities in the Prairie West District, and promised that she would contact the mental health nurses and social workers in the city. There was no set date for Kaija's release from the hospital, she assured me; it always depended upon finding a suitable placement.

Meanwhile, I visited Kaija in the Elliston Wing every second or third day. Each time I went with the secret hope that she would have improved and might be allowed to return home. But there were two obstacles to that. The first was Kaija's behavior. Each time I went, it was the same obsessive chant: *"I'm not admitted ... I'm not supposed to be here ... There's nothing wrong with me ... I'm going home!"* It was impossible to visit. One time she escaped out the door, spotted my car, ran over to it, and meant to get in. Fortunately, I had locked it. This deterred her not a bit. She just stood by the car and refused to move. I left her there and went back into the hospital, hoping that she would follow, looking for me. No such thing! After fifteen minutes of waiting and watching her from a hidden vantage point, I went back out to try to get her to return without having to call security. It began to rain, but even that did not faze her at first. Nevertheless, when the rain increased in intensity she reluctantly allowed me to lead her back inside.

The second obstacle came up unexpectedly. Dr. Ahmed had sent Kaija to an endocrinologist again, this time for a biopsy. Although the results showed borderline hypothyroidism (an underactive thyroid, Dr. Ahmed explained) just as the earlier blood tests had shown many weeks ago, he decided that he wanted to treat her for mild hypothyroidism, or Hashimoto's Disease anyway. This would mean treating her with large doses of steroids, Prednisone in this case.

Besides that, he had just started her on a second antipsychotic, Pimozide, and he needed Kaija either in the hospital or close by so that he could closely monitor the effects of both of these the drugs. Both sounded kind of scary to me; I knew that steroids played havoc with one's hormones and could have disastrous side effects if not carefully controlled. And when I looked up Pimozide on the Internet, the first thing I read was, "Use this antipsychotic as a last resource." I challenged Dr. Ahmed's choice of this, but was assured that "the dosage will be very small, only five milligrams to start with because we want to maintain the Zyprexa at its current level. Even though research shows no proof that using a combination of antipsychotics is more effective than just one, he reiterated, "Still, we've had some success with this and I want to give it a try."

What could I do but agree? Kaija would not be coming home.

One day, about two weeks after Kaija had been readmitted, I got a call from Glenda McKenzie. She gave me two contacts to call—one who could direct me to personal care homes in the city, and the other who could help me locate mental health care homes. I met with both contacts. I wanted to see the mental health care homes, too, in spite of what Dr. Ahmed had said. In some ways, I thought, they might be a better option because at least these caregivers would have had training in understanding and handling patients with mental illnesses such as Kaija had. And I wanted to find out if there were different levels of severity of illness that individual homes would accept.

Both contacts gave me a long list of addresses, and told me that it was up to me to contact the individual caregivers to set up an appointment to see the homes. Both assured me that I did not have to accept the first one that came available; I had to be satisfied with the home and I would have the final say on which one might be suitable for Kaija. They would let me know of each vacancy as it occurred.

At present, there was a vacancy at only one mental health care home. I immediately went to see it. There were five clients. None of them appeared to have severe psychoses, at least as far as I could see. The caregiver assured me that all were mild cases and easy to manage. But the rooms were all in the basement. It was dark and dingy. The windows were small and high up. I felt claustrophobic and knew that this was not a facility in which I could place Kaija. I called the social worker to let her know.

"That's fine," she said. "I'll let you know when others

become available. It's almost the end of the month, so some should be available soon."

Two days later she called again. "There's a real nice mental care home coming available in three days, on August 31. It's on a cul-de-sac in a quiet suburban neighborhood. I remember that the rooms are on the ground level and they're bright and cheery. And the caregiver is a real sweet lady who is very good with, and to, her clients. You should give her a call, because you don't want to pass this one by without seeing it."

The social worker was right – it was a nice home in a quiet cul-de-sac. Bonus features were the large, covered patio with comfy deck chairs, where Kaija could go to smoke, and a huge backyard with all kinds of shrubs and flowers and fruit trees, as well as a vegetable garden. The only drawback was that the rooms were shared, two to a room. However, the clients, all females of various ages, had only mild psychoses and all got along with one another very well. More important, Jan, the owner and caregiver, was not only pleasant but had twenty years of experience in her role and had earlier worked as an RN. I could tell immediately that she was an understanding and compassionate woman, and this meant as much to me as any other criteria.

"I'm not in a hurry to fill the vacancy," Jan told me. "I haven't had any other applicants yet. From what you tell me about your wife, I think she would fit in well here. Her roommate would be an elderly woman who is very quiet and mostly keeps to herself. If you wish, I can call you when I get another applicant, and give you first chance of refusal."

"That's awful good of you." She must like me or

something, I thought, to give me this option. "I expect that Dr. Ahmed will want to keep her in the hospital for a couple of weeks anyway, to monitor the changes in her medications. I'm still hoping that these changes will be significant enough that he'll allow her to come home again, even though he said, when she was admitted, that this was no longer an option."

"I hope, for your sake, that that might be the case. But remember, even if she does come here, it may be for only a short time. I've had some of my clients here for many years, but others for as little as two or three months."

I called the social worker to relay the results of my visit. She, too, promised to let me know if another referral came through her office in the next while.

It was only two days later, however, that I got a call from the social worker. "There's been another application for Jan's Mental Care Home. I talked with Dr. Ahmed about your situation, and he strongly suggested you take this placement right away. However, he recommended that Kaija go there for a three-day trial period, then come back into the Elliston Wing for an evaluation of the situation. Jan needs to get to know Kaija, too, and decide whether or not she's a client she'd like to have and be able to handle. The caregiver always has the final say."

"Well, I guess a trial wouldn't do any harm. Will they transfer her there directly from City Hospital?"

"No. It's up to you to pick up Kaija and take her there yourself. The staff has no jurisdiction outside of the Elliston Wing. And usually it's better if the significant other takes the patient and helps her to settle in. So, Dr. Ahmed said you can pick up Kaija from the Elliston Wing tomorrow morning and take her there. They'll have the paperwork ready."

"It seems like they're trying to get her out of the Elliston Wing in a big hurry all of a sudden. What gives? Do they need an empty bed for someone else?" I could not hide my sarcasm. It seemed like a paper shuffle or a chess game, but with humans instead of paper or pawns.

"No, that's not the case. Dr. Ahmed just wants this trial to happen now when there's an opportunity. That way he can determine whether this home is a suitable option. If it turns out to be so, you can always hold it with a deposit until he's ready to release Kaija."

No words could describe the heaviness of my heart. I hadn't anticipated such steamroller action. It brought me face-to-face with what I was actually engaged in doing—putting away my wife. It seemed such an irrevocable step, such a mean and dastardly deed.

My guilt overwhelmed me, and I spent the evening in self-recrimination and tears. Surely I could have coped with Kaija at home. Surely this new antipsychotic would work. Maybe it had all started with a thyroid problem after all and her psychosis would disappear in a few short weeks. I could handle her for that long, no matter what her behavior. I just needed more patience. I could get someone, anyone, even an au pair from overseas to help out. I loved her too much to let this happen. Hah! Let it happen? I was helping to make it happen!

This seemed like the first step toward separation forever. It seemed to me a mockery of our promise, "till death do us part." And now here I was, arranging what might be a physical parting for the rest of our lives.

It took all of my skill and energy to get Kaija just to

enter the mental care home the next morning. I likely wouldn't have succeeded at all if Jan had not noticed us, come out, and invited us in for a cup of coffee. We all chatted amiably enough at the coffee table, but as soon as she was finished, Kaija got up, stated firmly, "I'm not staying here," and walked out.

"I'm not staying here," she repeated as she went down the steps. "I'll walk home." And she proceeded to walk swiftly out of the cul-de-sac. I had to run to catch up with her.

"Come on, hon, you can't walk home. It's sixty miles and you don't even know which way to head from here." I stood in front of her, blocking her, holding her by the arms.

"Let me go. You're not putting me in there!" She struggled to get out of my grip and by me. "I'm going home whether you want me there or not."

"Listen, hon, this is only a pass for the weekend to see if you'd like to stay here instead of in that noisy hospital where you've already spent too much time. Since Dr. Ahmed won't release you to go home, I thought this would be a lot more pleasant option for a while."

I finally managed to restrain her and, holding her firmly by the arm, led her back. At the door, she suddenly grabbed the storm door handle with one hand and the wrought iron stair railing with the other.

"I refuse to go in there. If I go in, I'll never get out! You can't force me! Let me go!"

No matter how I tried, I could not pry her hands free. She blocked the entry with her body.

"Shut that door," she yelled at Jan. "I'm not coming in there!"

As we struggled, Kaija grew more and more upset, more and more angry and adamant. The scuffle brought a neighbor hurrying over.

"Do you need help? What's happening? Should I call the police?"

"No! We're OK. There's just a personal misunderstanding here, but we can sort it out on our own. Just don't bother us right now."

After about five full minutes, Kaija's energy began to wane and I was able to pry her loose.

"Please come in for a few minutes," Jan coaxed. "Let's go sit on the patio where you and Charles can rest and have a smoke. I won't lock the door; if you still refuse to stay after that, then I'm not going to try to stop you."

Probably it was the warmth and sincerity in Jan's voice that made Kaija acquiesce, but then again, maybe it was just the need for a cigarette that convinced her to go through the house and onto the back patio. We smoked. Jan brought us another cup of coffee. She talked to Kaija gently, not about staying, but just about her own life, her nursing career, her purchase of this care home so that she could stay at home, raise her two kids, and still have an income. She asked Kaija about her life, too, and they chatted amicably for ten or fifteen minutes. I just let them talk. I could tell that this lady was sharp. She related so effectively, yet still so genuinely to Kaija. Kaija warmed to her and was almost her normal, prepsychotic self.

Finally, we got up and I gently led Kaija to her designated room. She went quietly, like a little lamb. There was no fight in her now, just quiet resignation and a touch of fear. She looked questioningly into my eyes,

eyes that were full of tears. She seemed to feel my sorrow as well as her own, for she held my head in her hands as I wept and wept. As our tears mingled, we blessed one another and held one another as though we'd never let go. I kissed her good-bye and left. It was the saddest moment in our lives.

Chapter 22: Hope Springs Eternal

At Dr. Ahmed's suggestion, I did not go to visit Kaija during her pass at Jan's. I called Jan each day to see how things were going. Jan assured me that Kaija had been a model client. They had visited each day over morning coffee, sharing life experiences.

"I know a lot about you and Kaija now. She's one sharp lady! And you've certainly had some wonderful experiences together, living in the USA, Finland, and even China."

"Has she been upset and lamenting about being there? Is she mad at me for leaving her there?"

"Not at all. She gets up happy in the morning, comes for breakfast, goes out for a smoke, and then goes to her room to lie down. That's the only thing—she won't do anything but lie on her bed all day. She won't sit in the common room and watch TV or read or visit with the others. She's friendly with them, but has little to say."

"I'm not surprised. She never watches TV. We don't even have one at home. And now I think it would compete with the voices that are so constant in her head, and thus just get on her nerves. She never did anything in the hospital, either."

"Well, in spite of that, she fits in real well here. She's a really nice person and I know she would be just fine here."

I was relieved that Kaija had settled in and was not suffering, at least not obviously, from grief and despair. But because of Jan's final comment, I had a premonition that Kaija would have to return there after the weekend had been evaluated. Nevertheless I was shocked when I called Jan on Monday morning to arrange taking her back to the hospital.

"She doesn't have to go back. Dr. Ahmed called and said that since she was doing so well here—as I told him she was—he was releasing her to stay here indefinitely. He's already contacted the pharmacy to fill her prescriptions, and they'll be delivered here by suppertime."

"That bugs me! Why did Dr. Ahmed not call me? Surely I have some say in the matter. What about the evaluation he was supposed to do after the weekend pass? Some pass—a never-ending one!"

"Dr. Ahmed made it sound like it may not be for that long—two or three months, perhaps. And he set up appointments for me to meet with him every four weeks to report on Kaija's behavior and progress. She is supposed to accompany me, and he said that he would be contacting you to ask you to be present also.

"How is he going to monitor the medications, as he said he would?"

"I'm to call at any time and talk with his resident doctor to report any side effects. Her medications come bubble-packed so administering them will be an easy task. He sure has her on a lot of meds."

"I know. They keep trying one kind after another, and now she has those steroids for her thyroid on top of all the others."

"Well, don't you worry about a thing. Dr. Ahmed suggested you limit your visits for the first month so that Kaija will start to feel that this is home now. If you come to see her right away, it will negate this factor; besides, it will just upset her when you don't take her home. She needs to stay in a calm and neutral atmosphere for healing to begin."

"OK. I guess that's that. I'll call you every few days, but if anything changes, please call me immediately, at any time."

A new phase had begun in our lives. I did not like it one bit, yet maybe, just maybe this would be good for Kaija's mental state. It seemed, from talking with Jan, that she was not so uptight, so paranoid, so angry and resentful as she had been for so long now. Perhaps the peaceful atmosphere really did have a bearing on her state of mind and her behavior. I caught myself hoping, once more. Did I dare?

* * *

It felt like self-torture, but I waited eight days before going to visit Kaija at Jan's. They were long, empty days, similar to the many days and weeks Kaija had been in the hospital and that I had spent alone. The fact that she had fought so hard against entering Jan's Mental Care Home, and that I myself had used force to get her through the door weighed heavily upon me. Although by trickery and collusion I had forced her into the hospital those two or three times, I had never before used physical force. It was totally against my grain; I had always abhorred those who physically abused their spouses. Now I had joined them.

It was one thing to have Kaija admitted against her will to a hospital, for I saw this as an institution that provided help to the ill. But a care home did not have the same meaning and connotation to me. It was commonly held to be a "put away" place, a "get rid of" place, a "sanctuary" that provided relief not so much to the patient as (in this case) to the patient's spouse. I had had a hard enough time accepting that a care home for the elderly was necessary when my mother-in-law and later my own mother had been placed in one in Riverview. I admitted that their care had become more than my sister-in-law and my own sister were able to handle, that professional nursing care was necessary, that physically they could no longer be cared for by family. But even at that, I had not liked it one bit. Here they had remained until their deaths, loved yet neglected—not deliberately, but simply by the lack of daily connection that occurred. Family members had all visited frequently, yet what were an hour or two every few days compared to all the rest of the hours in every day? How lonely they must have been.

After a week I was an emotional wreck. I could stand it no longer, and so on the eighth day I went to visit my Kaija at Jan's. Her very rational behavior, her happiness and animation when I took her to supper at the Red Lobster reinforced my guilt. She need not be in here, I thought. There seems to be little wrong with her now. She speaks and acts so naturally, so rationally, so like her old self. This is crazy having her in a care home. Obviously, she's improved so much that she could be at home.

But my house of cards crashed when it came time to return to Jan's. Kaija was furious when I turned into the cul-de-sac. She refused to get out of the car. I sat with her for fifteen minutes, trying every way I knew how to get her to go in with me. I went into Jan's myself, hoping that Kaija would eventually follow me in. For twenty minutes I remained inside talking with Jan, but Kaija did not budge. Jan went to talk to her, but had no luck. Audrey, a friendly young patient, tried but again to no avail. Finally, I went to the passenger side door and talked to her both gently and firmly, but neither approach helped. When I opened her car door, she slid across the seat to get away from me. Once again I had to resort to force. I forcibly lifted her feet out of the car, bent her knees, put my arms under her shoulders, and lifted her out. She resisted it all, but had not the strength to match mine. With one arm tightly around her, I led her into the house.

For a few minutes, as we had coffee and a cigarette on the patio, she reverted to her pleasant self. But this lasted only until I said I had to leave. Then it was a reenactment of the many times I had parted from her in the hospital: anger, tears, the same old verbal abuse. *"You're in denial. You just want me to die,"* and on and on. She curled up on her bed and refused to say good-bye. In tears, I left her there, crying.

That night, I could have sworn that Kaija had crept into bed beside me, but when I awoke, I found her side of the bed cold and empty. Later the same night I was sure I heard her coming up the stairs. I waited, holding my breath in order to better hear her. She did not come. The next morning I felt as though nothing was worth doing. I wept. My body ached. I felt worn-out, and immediately after breakfast I lay down on the sofa and slept two hours. The day was heavily clouded, just like my mood. I forced myself to stay away another week. When I did arrive, Kaija met me with an astonished look.

"You got in this time! For six days you've been invisible and they couldn't let you in. Can we go home now?"

I stalled by taking her to Starbucks, picking up a grande bold coffee, and bringing it back to enjoy on the patio. She showed me about the backyard, commenting pleasantly, but in the middle of her chatter she said, *"Yesterday two jets flew over; they talked to me and I blessed them."*

"I wish I could take you home in one of them," I joked. "But I can't take you home today."

That started it: "I've been here for two weeks already and I was only supposed to be here for three days."

"You're right, hon. But Dr. Ahmed said he wanted you to be in the city longer so he can continue to monitor the Zyprexa and Pimozide for a bit longer."

"*Ahmed is not my doctor any longer! There's nothing wrong with me except my platelets ... You just hate me and don't want me home so you can run around and have fun.*"

"You know that's not true."

"I'm not going to any eye doctor or herbalist, either, like Jan said I have to. Just take me home so I can go see Dr. McRae, my own doctor."

"I can't, hon ..."

"Just go home then! *You don't even want to see me ... You're in such denial!*"

There were no hugs or kisses. Kaija went in to her bedroom in tears. I left, bitterly regretting that I had even come.

Ten days later Kaija refused to go to her appointment, so I met with Dr. Ahmed alone.

"Kaija is an enigma. We still can't figure out the causes of her psychoses and we're only treating symptoms. Her thyroid is not really abnormal, though the antibody count is a bit high. The MRI showed nothing. There may well be a genetic factor here, as you suggested earlier. She has a very strong personality—that's been advantageous in her life up till now, but now it's a detriment. That's one reason I want her to be in the relative seclusion at Jan's for a longer time, because there are no negative (or familiar) stimuli for her to react to there."

Against my better judgment, I stopped in to see Kaija. Of course she asked right away if I had come to take her home. But she did not become vehemently demanding or angry when I said I could not. Rather, she was relaxed and quiet, so I grabbed the opportunity to try to explain to her how things really were in our lives now.

"I'm not the one that's responsible for your stay at Jan's, hon. Dr. Ahmed insisted on it because he said you're not well enough yet to be at home, and the hospital atmosphere is not pleasant for you. This is much more peaceful. You need to accept that you're ill, darling. Your constant hostility and defiance are not your normal self. Your inability to concentrate and the times of confusion you complain about are surely signs of a mental health problem. The lies and the criticism you hear on 'ad lib' are not normal—you never had these before. You need to see Dr. Ahmed at future appointments so that he can help you get well. We need to face it, hon, you may be here at Jan's for a long time, perhaps a few months. Try to accept this for now and make life as happy as you can under these circumstances that God has placed us in. I'm as unhappy as you are about the situation; I do want you at home, but that just can't be right now."

To all this Kaija listened quietly, without any comment. When I stopped talking, she quietly suggested that I leave and go home. She expressed concern that I would not be able to see to drive because I was crying. This time there were long hugs and many kisses, and we greeted one another good-bye with God's Peace. Kaija stood at the door and watched until I was out of sight.

The next two visits, a week apart, went about the same. Kaija was more subdued, yet was full of hallucinations. When I phoned Jan in between, however, Jan told me that Kaija was sure that I had died. She checked the obituaries every morning to look for my death notice. Once she had explained that "*his liver exploded and he's in heaven.*" When I talked to Kaija on the phone and told her what I had been doing, she shouted, *"You're lying! You're in heaven."* When I had remonstrated that I could not be in heaven since I was talking to her on the phone, she replied, *"You're Mo. Charles is in heaven."*

* * *

I was becoming more and more emotionally unstable as time went on and it began to seem as though Kaija's stay at Jan's might be interminable. I could not stand more than a couple of days and nights at home alone, in a house that had become so, so empty. I took to going to my sister's and to Kaija's sister's for two or three days at a time. At one point I went combining canola with my nephew for a week. Driving his large, self-propelled John Deere combine helped; it forced me to concentrate on the swath feeding steadily into the pickup, leaving no room for rumination. The long days tired me out, too, and I slept soundly and peacefully each night. But when it was over and I returned home, I felt the loneliness all the more.

I wrote in my journal the next evening:

All alone again. I feel like I'm soon going to snap. Am so lonely tonight. So uptight, so strung up. Took an Ativan after supper. Hate this! Yet I can't always be perched at someone else's place. What a shabby life! No meaning. No drive. Force myself to do things: reorganize my pics on the computer, read easy-reading Louis L'Amours, Luke Shorts, Max Brands. These distract me for a while but I get antsy real soon and have to wander about, smoke, eat, try to nap, sometimes go for a walk, though I don't have the ambition for that.

My siblings and in-laws have all urged me to take a break, to get away, entirely away, somewhere. Where? To go touring alone is absurd. I'd only feel worse knowing that Kaija should be at my side. Besides, I didn't think I could handle the guilt of going off, supposedly to enjoy myself, and leaving Kaija behind, trapped in a care home, trapped in her mind, alone in a strange world.

One night my cousin Shandra, from Arizona, called me. "You should come and stay with us for a while. The desert sun will do you good," Shandra said. "You can just relax and soak up the rays while hubby and I go to work and carry on with our daily affairs. We won't bother you, unless you want to be."

So I went. Caught a flight south, hoping to escape for a week or two the never-ending stress, yet afraid that my guilt would shadow me day by day. Afraid that Shandra would be too busy, after all, to hear my personal lament. Afraid that it would have to stay locked up inside me.

"Oh, I'm so glad you came," she said, a genuine smile lighting her eyes. The hug was real, so I hugged back. It felt good. We had been close when Kaija and I had lived there for a few years, many years ago now. We had remained close, connected via telephone and e-mail on a regular basis.

"You can stay with us the whole time, if you want," she assured me. "But if you want to visit your other relatives and friends you can use our Ford half-ton. It's an extra, so come and go as you please—just leave time for me. I've taken some days off work here and there to make sure we have time together."

"I'd like that," I said. "I know it's good for me to be with people to get my mind off my sorrows, but I can't handle crowds right now and yes, I would like to spend a lot of time just reminiscing and visiting with you, if you're sure you can find the time."

"As a matter of fact, I'm going to be somewhat selfish about that. I really don't want to share you much at all, but ..."

"It's OK," I interrupted. "I'll visit later, but right now I need to lie low and I'm happy to spend the time with you." I couldn't explain how important that was to me, nor could I explain the tears I fought back. I only knew they were bittersweet. I had brought a lot of baggage with me, and now I felt that I could gently set it down.

* * *

Shandra was the same as I remembered her from earlier days: hyper and caught up in a rush of everyday activity. "After work I've gotta run and do some grocery shopping," she said the first day back in the city after a relaxing weekend at their cabin in the pines up North. "But then we can chat over a cup of tea as I make supper. Darryl—have you met him? —is bringing Suzie and

Dawson over so I can babysit them while they go to a Thanksgiving celebration at his workplace. I think they're such cuties, even though I'm a prejudiced grandma. But we can still visit later. They'll be back by 10:00 PM." And so we did, late into the night sharing memories of the good ol' days. But she had a listening ear and an empathetic response to Kaija's and my current problems, too. I told her everything, and as we talked, I experienced a powerful catharis. I suddenly did not feel as though the world had ended.

Tuesday was the same. "I've got to do hubby's payroll after supper tonight, but first I've got to shovel this place out. I didn't have time to clean before you came and this place is a disaster!"

"Don't you ever slow down?" I shouted over the roar of the vacuum as I came in from the back patio to grab another cup of coffee. It was relaxing to sit under the stars and watch the lights of the planes coming in across the valley. "You're always in a sweat over something. This place doesn't have to be spotless just for me."

"No, but it does for me! I'll join you in a few minutes now, but I just have to get to bed by midnight if I'm going to get through another day of work tomorrow."

"Tomorrow" was much the same. "I have to serve coffee after Bible Class tonight. Do you want to tag along, or would you rather just kick back here?" I went. I even enjoyed it a bit, chatting after the lesson with a few old friends.

Thursday provided some relief, for she took the day off just so we could hike Camelback together. We sat at the summit, gazing over the city and just chatting for over an hour. Later, we went to Starbucks for a latte, wandered through the Botanical Gardens, picked up some salsa for the Mexican supper she was planning, and stopped by her hubby's job to bring him a can of paint he needed.

"The kids—Dave and Julie, Mike and Peggy, and their kids are coming over to see you after supper tonight," she announced, clicking off her cell phone for the umpteenth time. "I told them they might as well come for supper."

"I'm making this baptismal gown for Jeremy and Shawna's baby," she said Friday evening. "I have to have it finished before Sunday 'cause the baptism will be here after church."

Saturday was simply a whirl. "I'll help you with your homework in a minute, sonny boy. Can you go get me a new toilet brush from Target, dear? Will you put on another pot of coffee, the strong stuff so coz here can enjoy it? I'm cooking your elk roast for you tonight, dear. Will you cut it while I finish this gown? Don't forget I have to go to my Curves class tonight, but I'll go after you get back from jogging."

And so it went, day by day for two weeks. Somewhere I lost track of her activities, yet I could not help but notice that most of her attention was directed outward. And she was in her element, doing what she enjoyed, expecting nothing in return.

But most of all, it dawned on me that she had time even for me. Perhaps especially for me. We visited many a late evening. She listened. I had a lot to relate and in between the frenzied pace of her activities she let me spill it out.

"It's OK to cry," she said, wiping tears from her own eyes. "You're going through a lot right now. I just wish there was some way I could help."

"You are, don't you know? I've needed someone to just listen for a long time. You've done that and more. Sure you've been as hyper as always, yet how many hilarious stories have you told me about your family, your grandkids, your work? How many past fun times have we shared so that we've laughed till we cried? That's helped me a lot. My sorrows have not been your sorrows, yet you've let me share my angst and lifted me out of my pain time and again."

And so she had. She was there, now, for me. She understood. She felt. She cared.

I knew now that when we went up to the cabin for the weekend it was for my benefit. I knew when she invited her married children and their families over for the evening that it was not to show them off but to bring me happiness at seeing them. I knew, too, that the taco salad, the enchiladas, the sockeye salmon, the sweet and sour spare ribs had been made especially for me.

And in spite of her selfish streak in wanting to keep me there, I knew that she had gone out of her way to see that I got to visit my other relatives and my closest friends.

She gave me life. She renewed my strength. I had found a soul mate. I needed that. I had sought it and craved it. Now I had it, and I cherished it.

As each day dawned and I ate my breakfast on the back patio, I let the early morning Arizona sun warm both my body and soul.

I renamed her in my mind: Angela Dawn.

* * *

I visited Kaija the day after I got back and told her all about my trip. She wasn't the least bit resentful that I had gone, and we had an excellent visit. There was no "Did you come to get me home?" There was no *"You're a liar."* No *"You're in denial."* No anger. No verbal abuse, aggression, or tears of frustration. Rather, she shed tears of joy at seeing me again. And I shed tears of joy, for the first time, when I had to leave. I was on cloud nine, even though in the back of my mind I knew this might be just a blip on the screen.

The next two visits, however, reinforced my optimism. I made a point of taking her out to better test how she was doing. Once we went to Olivia's Emporium for haircuts and an infrared sauna, then went to the Granary for a super good meal. Kaija was at her best, although her smiles disappeared as soon as I took her back to Jan's.

The next time, at Dr. Ahmed's suggestion, I took her to a hotel, the Western Inn, in order to get a fuller picture of her temperament and behavior. Mostly it went well, although every time I went to the bathroom, Kaija followed me and stood at the door *"so that you won't become invisible."* There were a lot of hallucinations, too, a few new ones but mostly repeats. But at no time did she become angry or demanding. When I told her I would not get "Jim Bream" for her, she did not argue.

Kaija had always liked hot-tubbing, so we spent a lot of time in the Jacuzzi and the swimming pool. I was horrified to notice, however, that Kaija had lost a lot of weight. I weighed her on the scale in the exercise room by the pool and was shocked. She weighed only 116 pounds! That meant that she had lost over thirty pounds over the last year, twenty of those since entering the hospital in

July. She had lost all muscle tone and looked very frail. I must have been blind not to notice such a great change before. I'd have to ask the doctor about that next time. Had he not noticed her weight loss? Was it the drugs that were causing this? Had her thyroid really gone out of whack these past few weeks? Wasn't she eating her food? Before we returned to Jan's, I stopped and bought two cartons of Boost. I asked Jan to give her one every day. She had been eating fine, Jan assured me, but she never ate sweets at coffee time as the others did. She, too, was shocked to learn how much weight Kaija had lost.

At our next appointment, Dr. Ahmed was not unduly alarmed at Kaija's weight loss. "Don't forget, she's a high metabolizer," he reminded me, "and such weight loss is often exacerbated by medications. It may have something to do with her thyroid problems, too, even though there is nothing seriously wrong there. But just high anxiety, which she suffered from July to September, would definitely have such an effect. Jan has told me that she smokes a lot."

"Yes, I know. She believes that she has to smoke thirteen cigarettes a day *"to stop her heart from vibrating."* She doesn't always sleep well, either, according to Jan. She's still going out for smokes at 10:30 and 11:30 PM, long after everyone else has been in bed for two or three hours. She has to get her thirteen in every day, about one every hour or so."

"Yes, Jan has told me about her sleeping problem, so I'm going to prescribe her Zopiclone, a sleeping pill. She can start on it tonight. How did your weekend at the hotel go?"

Dr. Ahmed was pleased with what I reported. "Do it

again in two or three weeks. She's settled in at Jan's well enough that you can start taking her out on passes every two or three weeks. But not home! That's out. It's not a neutral place, and she's not ready for that yet."

"What would happen if I just took her home some weekend? Not that I plan on it, but I just want to know what the procedure would be if I did so and then had trouble getting her to come back."

"That would be a bad move, because if you did so without a formal, written pass, I would have no authority to get her readmitted to Jan's, or another care home."

And so I took Kaija on another hotel outing midway through December, this time to a fancier one, the Parkland Inn and Suites. It was a much better weekend than the previous one. Whereas last time she had many hallucinations and fears, this time she expressed only four: *"Can you go pee? Lars won't let you ... Don't go to the car; you might become invisible ... The new lady at Jan's also 'ad libs.' We all do ... They have Jim Bream at the front desk, but you can't get it with Lars out there."*

My journal, written after I returned Kaija to Jan's and gone home told the tale.

> Kaija animated and alive most of the weekend. Loved the Jacuzzi and pool as before. Enjoyed looking at lots of pics on Bebo, and interested to see how the program worked. Really enjoyed the most excellent buffet in the hotel restaurant. Went to Sunday School Christmas concert Saturday eve. Was enraptured the whole time and kept asking me questions and commenting on performances. Commented on the good coffee each time I made it, twice as strong as the directions said. Actually read many articles in *Time* magazine, once for a whole hour and a half—a first! Was really interested in looking at pics and Xmas cards that

had come so far, as well as the album I had put together of all the pics taken of her in China.

When I took Kaija back on Sunday, I was bowled over by Jan's comment when I was talking to her alone: "I feel guilty taking your money. Kaija doesn't need to be here. She's been so much better lately."

At the debriefing with Dr. Ahmed at the next appointment, I was shocked again. "I'm going to give Kaija a two-day pass to go home for Christmas. I think she has progressed enough that we can try it. You'd like that, wouldn't you, Kaija?"

The biggest, sweetest smile lit up Kaija's face. "Yes," she simply said. The smile said all the rest.

"But remember, only for two days. And you have to come back to Jan's. Will you do that?"

Kaija looked directly into Dr. Ahmed's eyes and promised, "Yes, I will come back." No anger. No tears. Just so sincere! So rational! So happy!

I picked Kaija up at 9:15 AM on the twenty-fourth. I was happy, but nervous. Would she be as complacent at home as at Jan's and at the hotel? Would she remember her promise to go back to Jan's after Christmas? Only time would tell.

It turned out to be a mixed bag, but certainly much more positive than negative. We spent a cozy Christmas evening at home alone, at Kaija's request. It was actually my wish, too. I wanted to be alone with her and to experience the peace of Christmas with Kaija quietly by my side. We played Christmas CDs, read the Christmas gospel, opened gifts, snacked on some salty goodies I had made, and just sat and enjoyed the candlelight and the Christmas lights on our wee tree.

On Christmas day, Kaija at first resisted going to her brother Lars' family, but once there she enjoyed the afternoon of sauna, turkey dinner, and later dessert and coffee. We came home by seven thirty, though, because Kaija was worn out. Overall, it had been a very good day.

We visited my sister's family on Boxing Day. Kaija was preoccupied for two or three hours looking at Christmas cards and at her nieces' photo albums. At lunch and supper she ate heartily, chattered with nieces and nephews, and reminisced with them about the times they used to visit us when we lived on our acreage.

We left at 7:00 PM, in a flurry of good-byes, hugs, and kisses. Mine was an enforced happiness. The dreaded moment had come, the moment that had been at the back of my mind all weekend, the moment to return to Jan's. I had been a rat. Before we left to go to my sister's, I had packed Kaija's things and put them in the car trunk. I had lived through such moments too many times to feel assured that this time would be any different. Perhaps it would, but I wasn't taking any chances.

I flipped down the multi-door lock just before we reached the T in the highway. It was not suicide I feared, for she had never exhibited such tendencies. Besides, she knew and believed that there was no shortcut to heaven. Rather, it was because I fully knew the depths of her imminent despair. How could I know to what impulsive actions Kaija might be driven at the moment of truth? I sure didn't want her jumping out of the car at the corner and running into the dark night to try to escape the inevitable.

"Why are you turning this way?" she asked, a mixture of surprise and fear in her voice.

"Honey, you know we have to go back to the city. You remember what Dr. Ahmed said at our last meeting. You could have a two-day pass to come home for Christmas from Jan's, but you had to promise that you would come back. You looked him right in the eye and said, 'I'll come back. I promise.'"

"I am not supposed to be going back there! I'm supposed to stay at home! I don't need to go back there," she shouted, the anger and tears spilling out over the dash and whipping into my face. I couldn't help but flinch, even though I had feared that this was coming. Was it in my psychopathology course in college so long ago that I had learned about repression? It wasn't just a vague, abstract concept anymore. She truly was not conscious any longer of her promise to the psychiatrist.

"I was perfectly fine all weekend," her tears cried out.

She was right, or at least partially so. It had been a fine two days overall. Christmas eve together, just the two of us, had been intimate and wonderful, the best time of all. Christmas morning church, and then the afternoon at her family's had gone just fine, too. Of course she had not been her old bubbly self, but she now had a sweet, quiet, innocent way about her that I, and the others, enjoyed. She had joined in the conversation, not animatedly as before, but with genuine interest and rational responses.

It was all over now. Just memories—treasured memories—for me. In a way, I felt that these had been two of the happiest days of my life. She was home! Yet constantly lurking beneath the surface had been the bitter knowledge that this moment would come to end it all.

But I had to be honest with myself, too. All had not been perfect.

"Are you going to go and get me that Jim Bream for my platelets?" she had asked soon after we arrived home.

"Look, honey, we've been through this a hundred times before. There is no Jim Bream, and alcohol is the last thing the doctor would prescribe."

"You're in denial! You just don't want me to get better. My platelets are thirty-eight over forty-four and if they get to thirty I'll die. You don't even care!"

"That's not true, and you know it. But I don't want to hear about Jim Bream and this platelet issue anymore. You know deep down inside that that's not the issue. You yourself told the psychiatrist that you felt confused, that you couldn't remember things very well, and that you couldn't concentrate because of people yapping at you over 'ad lib' all the time." I had long since acquiesced to her insistence that everyone could talk on "ad lib."

"You just don't want me at home. I'm going upstairs to rest. *But I need to have my smoke first. I've only had five so far today and the doctor said I need to smoke thirteen a day because of my heart fibrillation."*

That had been the only off-the-wall outburst, a repeat of one of the recurring hallucinations over the past two years. But there had been other recurring lapses too—the lips moving as she silently conversed with the voices over "ad lib" and the initial resistance to going to her brother's: *"Lars is dead and Jean's gone to Washington. And how can we take Dad with us when he's already gone to heaven?"* she had said. Perhaps there had been other moments as well, but I could not remember them right now. Maybe I was repressing things, too.

I drove in silence through the black night for a long time. Finally, I could bear her weeping no longer. My guilt knifed into my side. Suddenly my own tears blinded me. I could see the road no longer. As I swerved toward the right-hand ditch, it was she who had the presence of mind to say, "You'd better pull over and stop till you quit crying." That was all. No sympathy, just a matter-of-fact statement. She let me hold her hand in silence after that. Resignedly she followed me into Jan's Care Home. I helped her unpack.

"I don't even have any cigarettes," she said.

"Yes you do. I brought four packs, and we left three packs here. You have enough for a long time."

"What's in that margarine container?"

"Just some of the home-baked treats we got for Christmas from our families. I put the ones that you like, the not-very-sweet ones, in there for you."

"Be careful driving home," she said. No longer any tears, no longer any smiles for me. Just a haunted look as she kissed me good-bye.

I drove off into the dark night, tears coursing down my cheeks, guilt stabbing at me incessantly. I didn't care if the speed limit was only ninety 90 km/hr. I stepped it up to 130. I had to get away, even though I knew that only a dark and empty house awaited me.

* * *

In spite of my deep sorrow and regret over what had just taken place, I soon recovered, for hope still lay strong within me. After all, I thought, Kaija's angry reaction to having to return to Jan's had been a natural, not psychotic, one. The taste of home must have been even sweeter to her than to me. I thought back over our two, or actually almost three, days together and decided that surely, in spite of everything, Kaija and I were still blessed. Kaija's candle of faith still flickered, that was obvious, and this had been so uplifting to me right from the very beginning of her illness. And our love, if anything, burned even stronger than ever before. We needed one another; we always had, but in a more poignant way now.

It was hope, however, that I found in the forefront lately. So often had my hopes been dashed that I learned to guard against them, to repress them so that my frequent tumbles into despair would not be so deep. But during Kaija's four months at Jan's, I had seen a real, measurable improvement. And Jan had, too, so it was not just wishful thinking on my part. Each time I had taken Kaija out for supper or to a hotel for the weekend, I noticed a significant diminishing of her hallucinations. And just as noticeable and important to me was that her disposition became so much more placid and bright. My hopes for a happy Christmas together were fulfilled. It had been a long time since she had been home—almost seven months. I visited Kaija each weekend in January, each time taking her out for supper or just for a drive to get her out of the house. I needed to test her response to returning to Jan's, and though it never made her happy, she had learned to accept it. Certainly her behavior was so much better than it had been for many months before her hospitalization in July.

My mother had often quoted, from where or whom

I knew not: "Hope springs eternal in the human breast." Only now did I fully grasp the import of those words. For the moment, even greater than love was hope.

"I hear you've been a good girl" was Dr. Ahmed's opening remark at Kaija's next appointment on January 22. "Is that true?"

"Yes, I've been good." A soft and innocent smile lit up Kaija's face. So childlike was her response that I marveled. None of her former discomfort and anxiety with Dr. Ahmed was evident. Nor was there any feeling that she was carefully responding in a way that would please Dr. Ahmed, or scheming what she should say to get released, as she had before. Pure and sweet—that was my Kaija!

"Charles faxed me and said your Christmas holiday had gone very well. How do you feel about that?"

"Yes, I enjoyed it. It was so nice to be at home again."

"Was Charles good to you?"

"Yes. He's always good to me."

"And were you good to him?"

"I don't know ... You'll have to ask Charles."

"She really was," I replied. "She was pretty upset about having to return to Jan's, but I can understand that."

"Yes. I talked to Jan a week ago and she told me she thinks that Kaija is well enough to be at home."

"I know. Jan told me she feels guilty taking payment for Kaija's care."

"Does that mean I can go home now?" interjected Kaija, gazing hopefully, and directly, into Dr. Ahmed's eyes.

"What do you think, Charles? Do you think she's well enough to be at home?"

"I do. As I've said in my faxes to you, it seems that the medications she's been on for the past few weeks are working much better than any she has been on before. Or at least that's what I attribute the improvement to."

"Jan told me that if I let Kaija go home, she'll hold the room for a month. She's going on vacation to Mexico anyway for three weeks, so she would not be taking on another client right away."

"Yes, she told me the same thing. She's very considerate."

"I'll tell you what I'll do. I'll give you an extended pass until the end of February. If all goes well you can stay home. But one thing you must promise me—that you'll take your medications every day and not stop them like you did before."

"I'll take them," Kaija interrupted eagerly. "I promise. Charles can give them to me."

"OK. Let's do that then. But I want to see you toward the end of February. You can book an appointment with the receptionist on the way out. Remember now. Be good to Charles, because if you are, I know he'll want to keep you there. And that's what I want, too."

"I hope Charles will let me stay. I promise I'll take my pills and be good. You'll see!"

* * *

And so, Kaija came home, once again, not for a fleeting pass this time, but hopefully, hopefully, to stay. As February came and went, she was as good as her word.

She took her meds from me, four times a day, without a single fuss; in fact, if I sometimes forgot to give them, Kaija herself would ask, "Will you get me my pills now?" She depended upon me so much now, and was so eager to please me. I was touched by her love—a tender, almost childlike love or, more exactly, a fresh blush of love such as we had known when we first met. My heart was full, every day. I felt her need and I responded with a pledge of servitude and a depth of love I had not known possible.

My hope was fulfilled, and Kaija's wish was granted. Dr. Ahmed allowed her to stay home. And as March passed and the soft spring breezes of April melted the frost, Kaija retained the state of equilibrium she had achieved while at Jan's.

The psychosis is still there. I have learned to accept Kaija's hallucinations as a normal part of everyday life. Almost daily she asks me to get her some Jim Bream, or some nonexistent pills for her platelets. Each day she is tormented by voices, especially in the morning and early afternoons.

"Lars is constantly nattering at me and criticizing every little thing that I do. He won't ever leave me alone. He keeps poking me all the time, too. He's just a flea with big glands!"

Indeed, I frequently hear Kaija weeping upstairs, and go up to comfort her. She will not give me any details when I ask what is wrong, or what Lars is saying. But always, just holding her helps.

As I hold her, I am fully aware that my arms encircle a wife who is far from being cured and who is still very ill. Kaija stays in bed upstairs most days. Some days she dresses, others not. I try in every way to draw her out, to entice her to do something. Sometimes I can get her to accompany me on a very short walk. She's frail and lacks strength—from inactivity, or mental stress, or medications, or perhaps all three put together. I do not know. At times I feel very frustrated, but I try my hardest to not let it show. Although I often have to fight off feelings of bitterness over the way our life has gone, I have nevertheless learned to curb my frustration and impatience so that it does not impact on Kaija. I have learned that people living with schizophrenia cannot tolerate strong emotion any more than one who has just come through a heart attack or recovered from a cancer operation. I have learned that alogia, or poverty of speech, and avolition, or lack of motivation, are common effects of schizophrenia. I long ago, after reading and reading, arrived at my own diagnosis: Kaija's psychosis was definitely some level, some form, of schizophrenia. I learned much from reading Elyn Saks' autobiography, *The Center Cannot Hold*, and the biography, *A Beautiful Mind*, based on the life of Nobel Prize winner, John Nash. I feel a strange kinship with them. They each suffered even more debilitating schizophrenia than my Kaija, yet each experienced recovery, to varying degrees, and each learned to accept and live with it. Kaija does not yet— perhaps never will—have such insight into her illness; she still blames it all on sticking platelets.

Yes, I feel I have learned much, both through study and through experience over the past twenty months. And the learning is still not over, I know. Kaija is still capable of surprising me almost every day. The wall separating reality and fantasy does not, for her, exist. It is like trying to draw a line in the water. It bothers me that she is so often entirely inaccessible, that she cannot (or will not?) tell me what is going on in her mind. She is still in lockdown mode. Her behavior, her expression, her emotional response or lack of it—in short, her entire illness—is just as incomprehensible to me now as it was in the beginning.

I still grieve the loss of my wife, the Kaija I was married to for forty years. She is gone, this Kaija who so enjoyed social activity, who loved her work in computers, who was interested and informed in all aspects of life. I rarely see the light in her eyes, the warmth of her smile, the joie de vivre that characterized her in the past. I truly miss her.

Yet, in spite of this, life is good. Although she has not the concentration to plan meals, Kaija often makes her own breakfast and lunch. She has begun to help me prepare supper and always helps clear up after. After resting for a while following supper, she often comes downstairs and spends at least part of the evening with me, reading, listening to CDs, looking at photo albums or our old scrapbooks, or just talking quietly and reminiscing. The past is important to her, and her memory is still 100 percent. This is fortunate, for in her present daily life there is nothing for her to talk about. Her conversations take place inside her head.

Neither memory nor faith have been touched by her illness. Although I cannot get Kaija to accompany me to church on Sundays, I know that it is not from a lack of faith but a fear of crowds. I am still astounded again and again when Kaija, after venting her anger at me during the day while in her other self (sometimes for not getting her Jim Beam, sometimes for reasons hidden within her psychosis), will, in the real world, come to ask my forgiveness an hour or two later. These are precious moments, when we can bless one another and again feel so lovingly close, so light-hearted, so free.

I have come to accept, albeit grudgingly, that our life will never again be what it was, that Kaija's recovery is relative and unpredictable, that the future is uncertain. But I am trying to achieve the patience to live just one day at a time. And I have learned to never give up on hope. I live for today and hope for tomorrow. Today I can hold my Kaija in my arms. I ask for no more.

And so I have made a point of being gentle with her. I no longer hope for a cure, but only a degree of recovery. Even this degree, at which Kaija is now, I am slowly learning to accept. I take comfort in my favorite Bible verse from Corinthians: "And now abideth faith, hope, love, these three; but the greatest of these is love."

I know it is true.

Wayne Kallio grew up on a farm in the Qu'appelle Valley near Tantallon, Saskatchewan. He earned a bachelor's and master's degree in English from the University of Regina, SK. He has taught high school and college English in Canada and Phoenix, AZ, and English as a Second Language in Finland, and China. He currently teaches adult classes in Special Education. He is a member of the Canadian Mental Health Association, the Saskatchewan Schizophrenia Society, and is a family member presenter in the society's Partnership Program. He and his wife Mary Anne live in Outlook, Saskatchewan.

Mind Gone Astray

Wayne Kallio provides us with a vivid, poignant and compassionate portrayal of his wife's roller-coaster ride with mental illness. The book conveys the day-to-day experience of psychosis from a spouse's perspective and how hope and love play an important role in dealing with the challenges of this journey.

Anita Hopfauf
Executive Director
Schizophrenia Society of Saskatchewan

Printed in the United States
140918LV00001BA/2/P